"In *Fit For Eternity*, clinical nutritionist and chiropractor Deidre Little presents a compelling recipe for healthy living. She uniquely combines candid sharing of her own weight and self-image struggles with her expertise in holistic health, but also shows clearly that the key ingredient is wholeness in Christ."

—Carrie Carter, M.D.

FIT *for* ETERNITY

DR. DEIDRE LITTLE

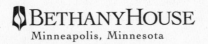
BETHANYHOUSE
Minneapolis, Minnesota

Published by Bethany House Publishers
A Ministry of Bethany Fellowship International
11400 Hampshire Avenue South
Bloomington, Minnesota 55438
www.bethanyhouse.com

Printed in the United States of America by
Bethany Press International, Bloomington, Minnesota 55438

Library of Congress Cataloging-in-Publication Data

Little, Deidre.
    Fit for eternity : balanced living through better nutrition and spiritual health / by Deidre Little.
        p.   cm.
Includes bibliographical references.
    ISBN 0-7642-2691-6
    1. Nutrition.   2. Nutrition—Religious aspects—Christianity.   3. Health.   4. Health—Religious aspects—Christianity.   I. Title.
    RA784 .L575 2002
    613.7—dc21   2002009660

DR. DEIDRE LITTLE, a speaker and a writer, is a certified clinical nutritionist and chiropractor. She has been the co-host of health and fitness radio programs and is president of Fit for Eternity Ministries. She makes her home in southern California.

The author's Web site is *drdeidrelittle.com*.

CONTENTS

FIT FALLACIES

Are you tired of the pressure to be thin? Forget about the pressure to be thin, let's call it the pressure to be perfect. Are you, along with much of our culture, tired of the fitness movement? Or are you becoming more desperate to attain physical perfection? The rise of obesity in our country may be a sign that we are overwhelmed, confused, and tired of being bombarded by diets, weight-loss schemes, and fitness. Everywhere we look we are faced with our inadequacies. Our society has so glamorized being thin that the insidious weight obsessions with which many are plagued have left most women feeling frustrated and ready to throw in the fitness towel. In some ways we've gone to the other extreme from the women's liberation movement. It's one thing to want the freedom to pursue a career but quite another to be enslaved to fit into a mold that sets us up for failure.

From magazine glamour to runway models, our view of what is beautiful and healthy has become very distorted. Surf the TV channels, and you will see station after station broadcasting the latest and best ways to take off those extra pounds in ten days or less. You can't even stand in line at the grocery store without catching a glimpse of magazine headlines proclaiming how you can have the perfect abs or buttocks in only five minutes a day. From pills and thigh creams to exercise equipment, there seems to be no escape. We are inundated with more information than we want. But have you noticed that the lines at the fast-food restaurants and donut shops aren't getting any shorter? The reality for most people is that they will never have buns or abs of steel; most are just hoping not to have buns of Jell-O.

For generations women have been influenced, even controlled, by what others have told them is beautiful, fit, and—for lack of a more suitable word—*normal.* Since society would like to dictate what is "normal" in every area of our lives, I challenge you to take a step back and think about how you've allowed society to mold your views of what normal really is. We have hundreds of diets, thousands upon thousands of pills and potions, all claiming to know the cause and be the answer. But do we really even know what healthy is and what it feels like? Or is "healthy" a feeling at all? How do we know?

> # Do we really even know what healthy is and what it feels like?

I believe it was Hitler who said, "If you tell a lie big enough and long enough, people will eventually believe it to be true." I call this the "Lullaby." In the "Lullaby," the devil is the wolf in sheep's clothing lulling the children of God to sleep through every method imaginable. He dulls the senses and mental clarity through an extensive campaign to take the nutrition out of foods but make them tasty and addictive to the point we would even fight for them. He dulls our sensitivity and compassion through violence in the media. He suppresses our immunity by bombarding our systems with toxic chemicals, medications, and excessive anti-biotics as well as with processed foods that are completely void of their original God-given nutritive value. He tries to wipe out our passion through perpetual opposition. He lures us into passivity, believing the lie that we few can't make a difference. He leads us to think that being pain- or symptom-free is equivalent to being healthy, so that we don't really know how to prevent problems.

We are fooled into thinking that living life fatigued is okay as long as we can have that cup of caffeine in the morning—even if it means standing in line for twenty minutes to pay $4 for a cup of coffee. Self-medicating (including common over-the-counter remedies) is big business. If we can self-medicate the symptoms of life's distresses, then we don't need to deal with the causes. After all, if it doesn't hurt, it doesn't exist, right? We have bought into the lie that superficial gratification is good as long as we don't harm anyone. Since the devil has made just about any pleasure readily available, we can justify our lust, laziness, and wastefulness.

We are now convinced that healthy and normal are subjective. But *common* is what most people really mean when they say *normal*. It is common for 55 percent of all adults over the age of 20 and 11 percent of adolescents between ages 12 and 17 in the United States to be overweight.[1] But it is not normal. We are so quick to say how someone suffers the *normal* weight gain with aging, has *normal* menstrual cramps each month, *normal* nausea with pregnancy, or acne, or headaches, or holiday weight gain. My all-time favorite is the oncoming "flu season." Since when did we add a season? There are four seasons: spring, summer, fall, and winter. For those of us who live in California, we basically have summer and fall. But "flu" is not among the "seasons." These things are not normal, though they may be common.

The first four definitions of *normal* in the *Merriam-Webster Dictionary* are

> 1: perpendicular; *especially*: perpendicular to a tangent at a point of tangency 2 a: according with, constituting, or not deviating from a norm, rule, or principle b: conforming to a type, standard, or regular pattern 3: occurring naturally <*normal* immunity> 4 a: of, relating to, or characterized by average intelligence or development b: free from mental disorder: SANE."[2]

Normal, according to Merriam-Webster, is based more on what is *not* normal rather than on what *is* normal. I find the first definition, "perpendicular," the most accurate. It most clearly matches God's Word: "For we dare not class ourselves or compare ourselves with those who commend themselves. But they, measuring themselves by themselves, and comparing themselves among themselves, are not wise. We, however, will not boast beyond measure, but within the limits of the sphere which God appointed us; a sphere which especially includes you" (2 Corinthians 10:12–13). The definition of perpendicular is "standing at right angles to the plane of the horizon: exactly upright." If the norm or standard is God's Word—our point zero, our horizon or true north in navigational terms—then anything outside of this standard is abnormal, though it may be common.

If the standard is based on the deviation and accepted as normal because it is *common*, it doesn't make normal any less true just because it doesn't occur often. But the Enemy has convinced us that the plumb line for mental health is the standard set by the psychologist; the normal for intelligence is set by the educators; the normal for spirituality is religious service or the maintenance of traditions; and the normal for physical health is set by the scientist. As far as appearance goes for women, we have believed the lie that unless you are thin, blonde, large-breasted, and blue-eyed, you are less than beautiful by the world's standard. "Barbie" has become the world's icon for beauty.

I will not be another author telling people how to get skinny. There is so much more available for us on this side of eternity, but if we are malnourished physically, relationally, and spiritually, we will not attain the power that is rightfully ours. I do see a change occurring. I see the pendulum swinging back from one extreme toward a more balanced stance. My suspicion is that the rise in obesity, heart disease, and stress-related illnesses in women has to do with their trying to assume a role not intended for them in society, while still trying to maintain a home, a job, and look like Barbie all at the same time. Normal should be based on God's Word—normal for our identity as men and women, normal for what is healthy, normal for what is moral and just, and most of all, normal for what is love in its fullest expression.

> ## God's Word tells us that the Word itself is our standard for normal in every area of life.

God's Word tells us that the Word itself is our standard for normal in every area of life. It tells us that the fear of the Lord is the beginning of wisdom, and that we will prosper in body and mind as our soul prospers (3 John 2). First Corinthians 3:19 tells us, "This world's wisdom is foolishness—absurdity and stupidity—with God" (AMP). In Genesis 1:26, God says, "Let us make man in our image," and He follows it by saying that what He made was very good! That means that every color of skin, every texture and color of hair, every shape of the nose, lips, and hips is good in His eyes!

But when man in his finite knowledge has taken what God made and altered it to suit his material, social, or financial tastes, distortion comes in. People would tell you, for example, that the adulteration of food is for our safety and for greater nutritional value, but, in fact, it is more to allow the "pie" to be cut into smaller pieces, allowing more people to have a bite. And I'm not talking about feeding the poor. I'm talking about the indulgence of the selfish rich to get richer at the expense of our health and emotional well-being.

For years I've believed Proverbs 31:8–9 is my mission: "Open your mouth for the dumb [those unable to speak for themselves], for the rights of all who are left desolate and defenseless. Open your mouth, judge righteously, and administer justice for the poor and needy" (AMP). Who are the desolate and defenseless? They are individuals who feel hopeless today. They feel that God has abandoned them. They feel trapped in bodies that are overweight and unhealthy. They are on the path to some disease and don't know how or what to do to stop it. Hell has had its grip on us for too long, impacting our health, and it's time to set people free. As the Lord warned Cain in Genesis 4:7, so He warns us today: "If you do not do well, sin crouches at your door; its desire is for you, and you must master it" (AMP). The door was opened years ago and Satan now stands unopposed and has full access to every area of our health. We have accepted this "Lullaby" as "normal" instead of what God's Word tells us is our heritage as His children (see Isaiah 54).

I will make no apologies. I firmly believe that in one way or another, directly and/or indirectly, sickness—disease (and that includes obesity)—is from the pit of hell. It is not normal, and its causes should not be tolerated. Hell has one purpose, and that is to separate God from His beloved. But as we, the saints of God, wake up and realize the tactics of our Enemy on every level, we can take back what is rightfully ours.

> **Every color of skin, every texture and color of hair, every shape of the nose, lips, and hips is good in His eyes!**

When we come to know Jesus as our Lord, our spirit is taken care of, but we have to live the rest of our lives on this side of eternity working out our salvation, healing the wounds of our past, and learning to love and to be loved. It's tough—impossible—in our own strength. But that's why I believe God said we are sanctified in spirit, soul, and body, because we need all three in balance in order to make it through "earth school" successfully. That's God's goal for us. Jesus told us that when we bear much fruit, we show and prove that we are followers of His and we glorify the Father (John 15:8). He wants us to be successful in the land of the living, not sick, tired—or sick and tired of being sick and tired.

Since the beginning of time humankind has eaten what God created, and it has provided all the vital nutrients needed to sustain life. But something happened. Just as we seek to understand what "normal" is, we should consider our understanding of what "healthy" is before we review what God did indeed provide for us to eat. When asked, "Are you healthy?" the typical answer is yes. My question is, "How do you know that?" Our answer is usually based on how we feel most of the time. According to the *National Vital Statistics Report* for October 2001, over 700,000 people died from heart disease in the year 2000, followed closely by cancer at just over 550,000.[3] It is a known fact that cancer can thrive in a person's body for years before the first sign is manifest to the individual.

Similarly, a person can have heart disease for 20–30 years before symptoms are revealed. For half of these, the fatal heart attack is the first symptom. Yet most people would say, "I'm healthy."

This tells me that our criteria for being healthy are not accurate. The dictionary definition of "health" is

> 1 a: the condition of being sound in body, mind, or spirit; *especially*: freedom from physical disease or pain b: the general condition of the body 2 a: flourishing condition.

I like this definition. It seems to fall in line with what Scripture says about being healthy, balanced, and sanctified—spirit, soul, and body. I would alter this definition just a bit. Freedom from pain is not always healthy, although no one would argue with the statement that a truly healthy person is rarely in pain. But let's look at a couple of possibilities where pain is not an indication of poor health.

A runner who takes on a few extra miles or a weight lifter who adds a few more pounds on the rack will experience pain with the increase in his workout. A mother who is delivering her baby will certainly experience considerable pain. What if you eat something that is tainted? You may experience considerable stomach pain and vomit what you ate. Is this a sign of poor health? No. The fact that your body recognizes the invader and eliminates it rapidly is a sign of good health. So what I would add to this definition is that health is resilience, the body's ability to bounce back when stressed or insulted with any emotional, chemical, biological, or physical entity. It also is the body's ability to quickly recognize harm or danger on these levels. Health gives the ability to live a long life with energy, vitality, mental clarity, strength, agility, flexibility, and peace of mind. Lastly, a healthy person will automatically maintain an appropriate weight for his or her height and frame.

Once we understand these basics, we can move forward on a firm foundation. In the following chapters I will share the lives of several different women, all of them beautiful in the sight of God. As you read, allow the Holy Spirit to do a work in your own heart to rewrite the scripts that have been embedded in you by an unhealthy society. Would you allow Him to write upon the tablets of your soul the original intention He had for your life when He knit you in your mother's womb? The Enemy does not have to reign in our lives. We know he is a thief, and in the power and strength of our Lord we can take back what has been stolen.

LIVING A FANTASY

We live in a fantasy that says if we follow ridiculous diets, they will actually bring about permanent, magical results; or even worse, we fantasize that the model in the ad will want to date us, marry us, and have children with us. The models we so aspire to be like have either worked very hard to get the bodies they have or they have eating disorders. But the point of marketing is to make us think we can be the person in the ad or be desirable to someone like the person in the ad. We want magic, not truth. Though there are numerous miracles recorded in the Scriptures, sometimes God works through a process, especially in the lives of those who are somewhat impatient. I would be a multimillionaire if patients could show up for an appointment, and *poof!* the weight would fall off by the time they left my office. Isn't that what most of us want—magic? And that's how many act—as though being thinner and healthier were a magical experience. The fact is, the average woman in America wears a size 16, and she didn't become that way because of one weekend binge on ice cream.

The fantasy I'd like to focus our attention on is the unreasonable expectations and pressures we place upon ourselves. When we buy into the lie, we become bogged down. Things become sinful when our confidence is no longer in Christ but is based on a distorted image. Weight loss and health goals are good as long as the lust of flesh, the lust of the eyes, and the pride of life don't accompany those goals. Philippians 3:3 tells us our confidence need not be in the flesh but in Christ: "For we [Christians] are the true ... who worship God in spirit and by the Spirit of God and exult and glory and pride ourselves in Jesus Christ, and put no confidence or dependence [on what we are] in the flesh and on outward privileges and physical advantages and external appearances" (AMP).

Are we rebellious, confused, or just stupid? I think I've been all of these at different times in my life. Why would anyone in their right mind CHOOSE to be obese with the known risks for heart disease and other inflammatory disorders? Not to mention generally feeling awful. For that matter, why would anyone CHOOSE to smoke with the known risks of lung cancer; speed and drive recklessly with the risk of an accident; do drugs while pregnant; drink while driving; and the list goes on. It's almost as though we are detached from reality and make choices with complete disregard for their consequences. Even the apostle Paul could not in his own strength control his behavior. He expresses with what I sense extreme frustration the disparity between his intentions and his actions: "For I do not understand my own actions—I am baffled, bewildered. I do not practice or accomplish what I wish, but I do the very thing I loathe [which my moral instinct condemns]" (Romans 7:15 AMP).

> The average woman in America wears a size 16, and she didn't become that way because of one weekend binge on ice cream.

I can't count how many times I have felt this way: I want to do one thing, yet I am driven to go contrary to what is good for me, blazing down the path the wrong way. Somewhere inside, we know that our destructive habits are not good for us; you can ask almost anyone, and she will tell you that she wants to stop but can't. Others will say they want to but don't know how. Many, unfortunately, say they would if they knew how, but when given simple tools, they find some excuse to not follow through. Of course, there are also those who really don't care.

The fact is, once we are given knowledge, we are responsible for what we do with it. True, we may be given wrong information. But if we are honest, we will find that we quit programs far more often than we find a program is not working. While we are on this earth, we have choices and responsibilities—as well as their consequences.

My hope is that you will be able to connect and maybe even discover your true self, your true purpose, and identify with the women whose stories I share in this book. You will then be able to decide if you have been rebellious or if you merely lack adequate information. Just as faith without works is dead, intentions without a plan of action are useless. I honestly believe that if most people could see clearly, they would choose what is good and right for them. But the Enemy of our souls has blinded many from seeing the truth. I recently heard a minister say that our prayers should be less focused on binding demons and more geared to having the spiritual blinders removed from our eyes. I feel this holds true for spirit, soul, and body wellness. If we could really see the truth, we would make healthy choices. We could get in touch with our true body image and stop comparing ourselves to the fantasy woman. Since I can't push a download button and instantly give you all the healthy living information that's in my brain, know that it's going to take time, effort, and determination—and the main ingredient is prayer.

HOW IS THIS BOOK DIFFERENT?

Because we are so bombarded with weight and health pseudo-solutions, I'm sure you are asking what is different about this book. First, it is not just another weight-loss book. Rather, it is a guide to being balanced: spiritually, physically, and emotionally. The benefit of being balanced is that you will reach and maintain a healthy weight. A balanced body will naturally reach its ideal weight. What I mean by this specifically is that when your body is getting all the proper nutrients it needs from foods and supplements, when it is eliminating toxins properly, when the digestive system is working properly, and the hormones are balanced, a healthy weight will be the body's natural response.

You may think such a result is impossible. I didn't say a balanced body would be *skinny*. I said a balanced body would reach its "ideal" weight. "Ideal" for a large-framed woman is different from what is ideal for a small-framed woman. We are

> Weight loss is—should be—the result, not the goal.

each unique and have different metabolic requirements. But I will say across the board that cellulite is not ideal and neither is obesity. Weight loss is—should be—the result, not the goal. The quest for the perfect weight-loss diet is futile. Because almost all weight-loss diets work, you may lose weight, but will you keep the weight off? Or more important, will the diet create other health problems? The quest for a balanced body, soul, and spirit will yield the results you really want. Yet the highest priority in this balance is your relationship with God.

I believe this is the first book to show how to take back what we've allowed to be taken away and to present a whole-person approach to weight management and whole health. I believe God initially gave the church responsibility for the entire being, not just the spiritual life. In Matthew 16:18–19, Jesus handed to Peter the responsibility of building His church. Over the years, however, the church has allowed its members to become fragmented. She has allowed the scientists to take the body and the philosophers to take the mind. She tried to keep the spirit but eventually allowed that to be taken as well. The bride of Christ was left a fragmented, torn, and bruised remnant of God's initial intention. But I know God wants His bride to be whole.

Obviously I am not saying we have to eat right in order to go to heaven. If you drive a Ferrari and put the poorest quality oil in it and never change it or tune up the engine, there is no way the car will run as well as the manufacturer designed it to. But it is still a Ferrari and always will be. Even if you wreck it, paint it, rip out the seats, and slash the tires, it will still be a Ferrari. Similarly, if you are a child of God, no matter what you do to your body, you will always be a child of God. But I don't believe a misused body is the Father's best for you. I want to help you to integrate your spirit, soul, and body so that you can be a whole, healthy individual.

Are you ready? As we learn who *He* is, He will show each of us who *we* are and how we can obtain true beauty. I know, because I was once that frustrated, weight-obsessed young woman. I was an inquisitive little girl bent on perfectionism. Eventually this self-induced pressure took its toll, leading to bulimia and years of struggle for acceptance and the perfect body. I was finally brought to my breaking point when the insanity of dieting nearly took my life.

The insanity of dieting nearly took my life.

Through my own journey and through journeying with my patients to be all God has destined us to be, I will journey with you as a friend who has "been there" but also as a doctor who has the tools to guide you. I can relate to the child who desperately wants love and attention. I can relate to the teenager who struggles with peer pressure, to the young professional woman striving for respect and success, to the single woman afraid of being left out, and to those women who just can't push themselves to enter a gym.

Have you left your first love? Life is so hard, and so often we turn to food for our comfort when life's pressures are overwhelming. Sometimes we make excuses that it costs too much to be healthy or it's too confusing, but really we don't want to know the truth because it will make us responsible. I understand because I was there. But God has given me not only the personal victory but also the tools for victory with my patients—and now with you. So get ready; take out your journal; come with me on this journey; you too can be fit for eternity, fully fit for the Master's use. Pray with me as we yield to the Holy Spirit for His leading:

Father, I come before you, hallowing your name. You are the God who sanctifies us; you alone are our shepherd and our peace. It is by your grace that we live and breathe and have our being. Because of your love for us, we have access to your throne of grace and humbly submit our heart's desires to you. Your will be done as you lead us into a healthier, more balanced lifestyle. We know that you are our healer, and no matter what we do, you alone are God and the creator of all things. Lead us as we consider the suggestions presented in this book and illuminate us by the power of your Holy Spirit. Make us all we were designed to be. Let your light shine in those dark areas of our lives; give us eyes to see where we have been misled or deceived by the Enemy. Give us courage to change and the confidence that you will lead us every step of the way. In your Son Jesus' name. Amen.

And may the God of peace Himself sanctify you through and through—that is, separate you from profane things, make you pure and wholly consecrated to God—and may your spirit and soul and body be preserved sound and complete [and found] blameless at the coming of our Lord Jesus Christ, the Messiah.

1 THESSALONIANS 5:23 AMP

FIT TIP #1:

Buy a journal—a pretty one, one you will enjoy picking up on a daily basis. When I see beautiful journals, I often buy them in bulk to share with others. There are so many choices. Each person has her own preference. Treat yourself.

1

FITTING IN

Perfectionism and Obsession

Who would have thought that wanting to be "fit and trim" would almost take my life and cause me to nearly lose all I had worked so hard to build? As I stood at the bathroom sink, I looked into the mirror, horrified, and vowed I would never throw up again. This was not a time to reflect but to decide. How would I handle the rejection, my fears of failure, and my desperate need to be perfect and not allow these feelings to control me? In the past I had secretly made vows that I would be forced to live out. Vows in which I said, "I'll prove those kids wrong who hurt me, teased me, and played dirty jokes on me. I'll become rich and famous. I'll show them they were wrong about me."

This Saturday afternoon, though, it was hard to focus on the truth. The lingering hurtful voices from my past spoke louder than the truth. The pressure to fit in and be accepted by the "in" crowd was so heavy on me that it drove me deeper into compulsiveness the more I was ridiculed and rejected. I didn't realize the reason my classmates were so mean to me had nothing to do with the truth. I doubted everything my parents said, including that they loved me, and I began searching for acceptance and "true love."

Though my parents continually told me I was smart, pretty, loved, and could do anything I set my mind to, the antagonism from the kids at school imprinted another message on my mind: that I was not smart, not pretty, and definitely not accepted. I tried so hard to fit in. I remember even trying to use curse words because it was cool. They just laughed at me. My pursuit for acceptance and "true love" proved futile and painful as the years went by. I worshiped daily at the "temples" of physical and mental perfection. Excessive exercise and dieting were commonplace in my everyday life in order to maintain my sanity, feel somewhat good about myself, and maintain control of what was around me.

My endeavors led to years of heartache and physical brokenness. At twenty years old, I was crumbling inside—until this particular afternoon: as I often did after bingeing on an enormous amount of junk food, I had knelt over the toilet and purged my shame. But this time was different. I'm not sure if I blacked out, but when I opened my eyes, there was blood and vomit all over the bathroom walls. After I cleaned the bathroom, I realized this was not a healthy habit, and it needed to stop.

Though I didn't have a personal relationship with the Lord at that time, I'm sure He was saddened by my desperate pursuit for love, acceptance, and perfection. I imagine He was calling my name, standing with open arms, as I wandered, looking in all the wrong places. My best friend from high school had already come to know Jesus as her Lord and tried to introduce me to Him. Funny, but I thought since she wasn't any good at geometry, how could she know anything? I ignored her introduction.

The Father longed to have intimate fellowship with me. He desired for me to know Him, to be known by Him, and to manifest the fruit of abiding in Him. "When you bear (produce) much fruit, My Father is honored and glorified; and you show and prove yourself to be true followers of Mine" (John 15:8 AMP). "Whoever lives in Me and I in him bears much (abundant) fruit" (John 15:5 AMP). Yet I was not aware of His great love, nor was I listening or interested in Him. The only fruit I was producing was self-serving and temporary.

The sad part of this is that I never shared how I was feeling with anyone. I suppose I felt it was so evil that my parents would think I was crazy. I held the shame inside, and until recently never told a soul.

Although after that horrifying afternoon I vowed never to purge again, over the next ten years I resorted to exercising excessively. I would wake up at 5 A.M., run three to four miles, then go to the YWCA to swim a mile. Then I'd go to school for seven hours, study, and go to the gym and ride the Lifecycle for an hour before going to work as a cocktail waitress until 1 or 2 A.M.

In addition to that insanity, I went on the watermelon diet, the lemonade diet, the grapefruit diet, the high-carbohydrate diet, and the low-fat diet, along with numerous "quick fix" weight-loss herbal diet programs. I tried colonics, fasting, and any concoction anyone said would keep me thin. Unfortunately, they all worked. Mind you, I am 5'7", and at that time I wore a size 4. Perhaps if I had been able to talk to someone, I might have been spared the destruction I inflicted upon my body. But I just couldn't. I believed the lie that I could not trust my parents, and I certainly could not trust those who tortured me. I had no one but myself to trust.

> In addition to that insanity, I went on the watermelon diet, the lemonade diet, the grapefruit diet, the high-carbohydrate diet.

HOW COULD THIS HAVE HAPPENED TO ME?

Looking back, I grew up in a home where I received plenty of love and attention. I remember the many times my dad took me to fly kites, to fish, or to play tennis. Mom loved to "make things pretty" and enjoyed hauling us kids around to visit and go shopping. My younger twin brothers and I enjoyed a typical sibling relationship: I tormented them and they harassed me. The tomboy I was preferred to either play football with the boys or stay inside and study. I wasn't too interested in the more "feminine" pursuits and was quite upset when I wasn't allowed to play on the boy's Little League team. I loved school and was a bit obsessed with the pursuit of knowledge. Actually, I was obsessed with just about every activity I undertook. My parents would encourage me to strive to do my best versus striving for perfection.

What seemed like a healthy childhood was marred by my interpretation of love. I believed the lie, as so many young girls do. I believed I needed to be and do certain things in order to be loved and accepted, and it drove me to a complete and total obsession with food and my weight.

When I was eighteen I had a modeling job that brought me closer to using food to feed the baby monster within me. If low on my measurements, I would eat a whole pie to gain a pound or two. Food soothed the stress of my school and everyday life demands. I couldn't handle the possibility of gaining any significant amount of weight, so I began to purge. If I didn't measure up, I wouldn't work. Combining this with the need to be the perfect student and the perfect daughter, I began to internalize this perfectionist pressure, and binge. I *never* felt good enough. My self-image became so distorted that I would look in the mirror and no longer see myself—just a fat person, and I would fall on my bed and cry. Food became my comfort, my compromise, and my enemy.

> I would look in the mirror and no longer see myself—just a fat person.

One morning when I was twenty-five years old, as I worshiped at the local temple of the perfect body—the gym—I met a man who was absolutely gorgeous. We talked, and he asked me to lunch. Lunch turned into dinner and dinners turned into a relationship. Though he was a Christian, he was not a godly man. But God had plans for our meeting; He wasn't going to let another year go by without my encountering Him. One afternoon my friend asked me about my life and if I was happy. I shared my academic and professional endeavors and goals. Again he asked me if I was happy. I began to cry, and then he introduced me to Jesus. Ironically the relationship ended that very week, but my relationship with Jesus began. I felt hurt and rejected, but I had a new hope in Christ and longed to know more about Him.

Jesus had a lot of work to do in my fragmented temple. Having just opened my first nutrition clinic, I had become a workaholic, high-stressed individual, who now tried to fit God into my organizer. I worked hard and was very successful in my practice in Los Angeles. I loved and lived my work, and it was extremely fulfilling. I enjoyed my time with the Lord, going to church and fellowship, but I had not fully surrendered my all to Him. My package looked good, but there was something missing on the inside. I was still striving to be perfect, loved, and accepted—even by God.

A DEVASTATED METABOLISM AND IMMUNE SYSTEM

Little did I know that all of those crazy diets and my insane lifestyle over the years had destroyed my metabolism and my immune system. Add a new business, a broken engagement, and a tenant who refused to move or pay rent for several months, and I entered the squeeze. I recently heard someone say, "Some people, you squeeze 'em, they fold; others, they focus." In my squeeze, I chose to focus, but it was very difficult.

I entered the squeeze at thirty-two. First, a severe kidney infection required hospitalization. A few years later I got pneumonia. This was truly the most painful experience of my entire life. For the first week the doctors could not figure out what was wrong with me. I remember nights of screaming in pain and finding no relief with the medication. They ran tests for everything from AIDS to Valley Fever and finally settled on pneumonia. My symptoms had followed a water-skiing trip up the Colorado River and began like the flu. But it wouldn't go away. Days turned into weeks in the hospital with a fever that would not drop, a month and a half in bed after that, and another two years with recurrent upper-respiratory infections.

The financial losses coupled with the loss of my pride led to severe depression. I had to keep working in order to survive. I gave up my home, my new Mercedes, and my confidence. I recall walking home from work one rainy afternoon: I began to cry and wonder what had happened to that successful doctor who hoped to do great things. I wondered what would happen to her now. Would she become a homeless person, standing on the corner talking to herself and shouting rude remarks to passersby? I had lost everything, even my hope. I felt God had abandoned me. After my breakup with the person I thought was the love of my life, my grandmother's death, the loss of my home, and my business decline, I felt like a lost puppy. My parents had been so proud of their successful doctor daughter. I was so ashamed that I had let them down and—worse—that the kids at school had been right; I was a loser.

But God was to prove me wrong. His healing way, though a long process, has shown me that I am valuable and that He loves me with all my imperfections. First, He healed me of bulimia. Though I physically stopped

I began to believe God had a purpose for my life.

purging at age twenty, the spiritual and emotional healing continued over the next five to ten years. I began to believe God had a purpose for my life. There was so much more to work through, but this was a huge breakthrough for me.

One day as I read Mark 11, I was struck by the words "He was hungry." These three words would not leave my thoughts. How could Jesus be hungry? After all, He could feed five thousand—couldn't He feed himself? There must be more to this. Mark states, "Now the next day, when they had come out from

Bethany, He was hungry. And seeing from afar a fig tree having leaves, He went to see if perhaps He would find something on it. And when He came to it, He found nothing but leaves, for it was not the season for figs" (11:12–13). Imagine Jesus' frustration. Having just experienced His triumphal entry into Jerusalem as the Messiah, He leaves Bethany with a certain degree of expectation. I imagine He was expecting the fig tree to be fruitful. But there was nothing. I wondered, *Could the fig tree actually be indicative of those who are supposed to be Christians? Was Jesus now looking at me, hungry for intimacy but only finding barrenness?*

My own attempts to fix my life had produced temporary results, but for the most part they had been futile. As I tried to make myself and my life perfect, I read and meditated on Colossians 2:10: "You are [I am] complete in Him [Jesus Christ]" (bracketed words added). I could not fix myself without first realizing that I was whole and complete in Jesus Christ. Only He could heal me and restore my life to health and wholeness. My attempts only brought frustration and disappointment to the Lord. I knew that apart from Him I was nothing and could do nothing of true worth and everlasting value. All the control I thought I had was nothing compared to the ability and willingness God had to truly change me.

"You shall love the Lord your God with all your heart, with all your soul, and with all your strength" (Deuteronomy 6:5). "You shall love your neighbor as yourself: I am the Lord" (Leviticus 19:18). It had become very clear to me that the greatest command the Lord gives us is to give ourselves to Him with all our heart, mind, soul, and strength. That meant that I was to love Him with my thoughts, desires, feelings, actions, emotions, eating, exercising, and view of myself. And second, I was to love my neighbor as myself. If I didn't love myself, how could I love my neighbor? If controlled by my emotions, experiences, upbringing, relationships, fears, trauma, and how I had responded or reacted to those situations, wouldn't this determine who I was and who or what I loved? These things had molded my self-image and either empowered or disabled my ability to love others and myself.

For me to be bondage-free and live a victorious life, I needed first to really know who God was, what He said about me, and what He wanted of me. Then I needed to do whatever I was told to do to have these traits expressed in my life. Only then could I without compromise love the Lord my God with all my heart, with all my soul, and with all my strength, and love my neighbor as myself.

Living fully in the balance of wholeness spiritually, physically, and emotionally is accomplished through understanding our identity in Christ and the willingness to see the areas that hinder us from becoming the person God intended us to be. To me, this is the divine design. To be transformed into the image of Christ is to know Him and learn who we are in Him. To be thin might be wonderful, but to be healthy and effective in one's life is powerful. When we are aware of who we are in Christ, our lives will manifest the fruitfulness of God's Spirit. Jesus hungers to have intimate fellowship with us, to produce fruit in our lives. This is how we glorify God and show that we are His followers.

ALLOWING GOD TO HAVE HIS WAY

A number of years have passed, and Jesus has graciously healed me of the symptoms of my eating and image disorder. Yet I have sadly experienced the consequences of my ignorance. Through anxiety and chronic stress in my life, I suffered a compromised immune system. I cannot emphasize enough how important it is to allow God to have His way. I believe God's Word that says healing is for today because He has not changed. Yet He allowed me to suffer the consequences of my actions because it was the only way I would listen or truly get to know Him. I struggled for years and shed many tears, not wanting to let some things go.

In my heart and in my words, I was feeling and saying that I was giving it all to God, but my behavior and the things that consumed me revealed a heart that was not fully submitted. I seemed to have peace as long as I had visible hope that my life was on track. When my business schedule was full, I had money in the bank, and someone was calling to say he was thinking about me, I was joyful. But if there was a lull in any of these areas, I found myself wringing my hands, wondering what I had done wrong, and wondering where God was. I still maintained a level of struggle or fear in my life. I still suffered daily with a degree of despair that I could not shake. I still wondered what I had done to deserve God's heavy-handed discipline.

> Even though I taught others the truth, for some reason I didn't believe it applied to me.

I battled with my understanding of God the Father. I still viewed Him as the heavy-handed disciplinarian. Even though I taught others the truth, for some reason I didn't believe it applied to me. My life was still one of struggle and continual striving over one thing or another. I did not manage my stress and anger well, and it would soon show. Whether it was to be the perfect daughter, the perfect doctor, or whatever role I was in, I lived by rules, not relationship. I lived by the perceived high expectations of my family. I had a good diet, exercised just enough, and did all the "right" things, but I lacked the key elements of the Christian life: joy and intimacy. At the onset of writing this book, at forty years of age, I was diagnosed with breast cancer. I was so tired and worn out, and as I stood in the shower one morning, I felt that still small voice of the Holy Spirit ask me, "Do you want to live?" Something inside of me rose up with the knowledge that I had a purpose that had not yet been fulfilled. So my answer, regardless of how I felt, was "Yes, YES, FATHER, I want to live!"

I know there are many women like I was who are trying so hard to live right before God, but who are living joyless, rigid, fear-filled, rule-bound lives. *Cancer* is one of the most frightening words anyone can hear coming from a doctor's mouth. Yet when I heard this diagnosis, I recall sighing with relief. It was as if I said, "Finally, I can get some rest!!" I was worn out and ready to quit.

I have endured many trials, and the powers of hell have tried to wear me out, tear me down, and shut me up. But God has planted a word in my spirit that I am committed to getting out. There have been seasons when I would have given up. But God by the power of His Spirit has risen up in my brokenness and reminded me that He has a plan for my life, and it will be fulfilled if I don't quit. So when asked if I wanted to live, I had no choice but to say yes. My life is to be poured out for the message placed within my soul for the purpose of building up the body of Christ.

As the father in the parable of the prodigal faithfully, daily looked for his wayward son's return, God the Father was waiting every day for me to run out of "me" and return to His house. He had given me so many gifts that I gratefully received, but deep inside I believed it was my hard work that brought my apparent success. Even though I verbally gave God the credit, I felt that if I dropped the ball, I'd lose the game. These gifts needed first to be acknowledged as from God and then to be surrendered daily to Him, to be filled with His purpose and renewed by His fellowship and intimacy. I knew these things, but I couldn't cross the chasm created by my fears and intellect. As he did with Gomer (in the book of Hosea), the Father had to lure me into the wilderness and speak tenderly to me. He allowed me to be stripped of everything the world had given me so that I would know it was He who had provided for me all along.

I felt like a character out of a movie. One day I'm worried about who's staying on track with their appointments, what supplements to order, or what color I'll paint the kitchen, when out of nowhere the plane of my self-important, mundane existence crashes, and I swim ashore "Cancer Island." Life really takes on a different perspective from the shores of Cancer Island. There are things that Gilligan never told us. It no longer mattered what color the kitchen would be or who needed an appointment. Everything stopped. Business, relationships, social engagements, producing, making a difference, all seemed to cease—at least to the degree I had known them. The shocking reality to me was that my lack of fear was not because I had the peace of God. I was just so worn out from struggling for so many years to "make it" that I would have happily surrendered and died.

Yes, I had some successes, and I had some good relationships, but life had just been too hard for too long, and I had no joy. It was at that point of revelation that I was really born again. I finally died and gave up. In the midst of it all, I had literally hundreds of people sending me cards, gifts, flowers, and books. I felt frustrated when people said they were praying for me. I thought, *Why bother, God has allowed this final blow to take me out. This has been one big joke, and the big guy has finally won.*

After months of chemotherapy, thousands of supplements, and numerous homeopathic remedies, followed by radiation therapy, the Father met me with open arms and compassion. Every area of my life had now been exhausted. Every

> The Father met me with open arms and compassion.

resource was gone. All that was left were Him and me. My body broken, my heart and spirit crushed, the Master Physician began to work on the root of the cancer. After years of striving to have the perfect body and the perfect life, I believed the lie of the Enemy that said I had to work hard to have a fulfilled life. Through this cancer, the Father gave me His love, and I could finally receive it and know I didn't earn or deserve it. He split the sky and reached into my broken life and provided for my every need in a miraculous way. He revealed himself as my provider, protector, healer, a fire by night, and a cloud by day. In the process, the scales fell from my eyes, and I was finally able to see Him the way He wants to be seen and known. And the amazing blessing was that He, the Father, the originator and creator of the universe, took away my struggle and blessed me with joy unspeakable. I am His beloved. I am radiant with the beauty of His glory within me. I am an heir of His inheritance, and that inheritance is God himself. He set me free to have true intimacy with Him, free from hiding, comforting my flesh with work and anything else that would temporarily remove the "angst" of feeling that I had to do it all on my own.

My only joy had been my work, and when someone was unhappy with me, I became depressed and felt like a failure. Taking everything personally makes life's burden really heavy. Even though I had not thrown up a meal in nearly twenty years, I had not changed; I had simply switched to a less life-threatening form of addiction. Unfortunately, the impact on my immune system was probably just as bad or worse. I was fooling myself into thinking all was well and that someday I would be happy, when my Father held the keys to joy in my present as well as in my future.

THE FATHER'S HEART FOR HIS CHILDREN

I set out to share with you what I feel is in the Father's heart for His children. Many of my sisters and brothers are living today in "struggle." Many struggle with their weight, while others struggle in their work, their relationships, or simply over what tomorrow may bring. But God the Father has poured out His love on us, and He has made provision to remove the struggle. Why? So you can get the guy, look and live like a supermodel, have a ball? No, He has provided a way to remove the struggle because He knows it holds us back not only from our divine destiny but also from the deepest form of intimacy possible—a relationship with Him.

In Luke 15:11–24, the Lord Jesus shares the story of a son who had spent everything, who struggled with life, thinking that his inheritance would bring him greater fulfillment and joy than he had living under his father's roof. He believed the lie—just like I believed the lie, and just like Eve believed the lie: that God is holding out on us, that we'd be better off on our own. But you need to know that any life outside the Father's house is a life of struggle and striving. All we have to do is "come to our senses." Unfortunately for most of us, this often occurs in the midst of a tragedy. Then we come to the end of ourselves and turn our hearts back in the direction of the Father's house. That's all we have to do, turn in that direction. He meets us on the road. Remember, the father in the story was walking daily out onto the porch, down the driveway, looking down the road to see if that day his son would be coming home. That faithful father saw his prodigal son a long way off and *ran* to him, throwing his arms around him, kissing him warmly. This is exactly what the Father did as I was immobilized after surgery. My heart turned a little toward Him as I experienced His love first through my family and friends. Day by day and week by week, I began to experience His love in deeper and deeper ways. Leery of His intentions and still not trusting Him totally, I watched and waited to get slammed, as I thought I had so many times before. This never happened; I only experienced His love. He ran to me and swept me up like a dancer in a beautiful ballet.

My surrender to His love occurred the morning I woke up, took a shower, washed my hair, and knew it was the last time for a while that I would be washing my hair. Talk about a bad hair day. It was like lifting a hat from my head, as all my hair fell to the floor. I cried as my parents hugged me, but I already had peace about it. I took the electric razor and shaved what remained of my hair and made my way to the wig store. It was my last nemesis. I had already had the surgery—the lump, plus surrounding possibly cancerous tissues had been removed—and now my hair. I felt ruined, spoiled, no longer beautiful. Overall, physically, I felt good through the entire ordeal. My herbs, supplements, and homeopathy worked very well. Of course, it was the prayers of the faithful even when I felt faithless that not only made the remedies work but also changed my heart.

There was a part of me that floated away that day my hair finally fell out. It was my last bit of control over my life, and as my hair was thrown into the trash bag, I saw a new identity begin to emerge: one that recognized that I was beautiful whether I had hair or not. When something like this happens, you come face-to-face with your true self-image. I realized I was beautiful even with a scarred breast and with radiation burns that left their insignia. God revealed to me in the most awesome and faithful ways that He loved me and that He would prove to me that I was loved, valuable, and—best of all—that I was His daughter, whom He would protect, provide for, and heal. He removed the emotional cancer of struggle; the lie the Enemy had fed me for so many years. It was finally gone.

> The book you are reading is not only about weight management but is also a love song of the Father to you, His child.

The book you are reading is not only about weight management but is also a love song of the Father to you, His child, to turn your hearts in the direction of home, because He is waiting, peering off the porch, looking down the road to see if you are looking His way. And He will be running to sweep you up into His arms and take away the struggles in every area of your life where you are willing to look in His direction. Whether it is your health, your weight, your emotions, your work, or something else, He wants His children *Fit for Eternity* and fit for His purpose.

In my practice as a clinical nutritionist, I enjoy seeing the transformation that God makes in patients' lives. Daily women come in wanting that quick fix. I could easily provide this, but what a blessing they would miss. In each face I see the fear, the yearning, and the hope. I have to tell them the truth and give them the opportunity to experience the true "fix" that only God can offer. I see Him turning over the tables of compromise and setting them free. Yes, practically we work through diet and clinical issues, but I know and I share that the true Physician is the one doing the real work, if we let Him.

I ask you, have you been searching to satisfy your emotional turmoil and inner cravings with food, shopping, sex, or exercise? If Jesus were to look at your life, would He find a barren fig tree? Who have you been trying to please? What lies have you believed? What truth do you know about how the Father sees you and feels about you?

Father, I thank you that you co-labor with us in our transformation. We desire to live a fruitful and victorious life. By the power of your spirit, we ask you to show us your truth and help us to be honest with you and with ourselves. In Jesus' name we ask these things. Amen.

Now may our Lord Jesus Christ Himself and God our Father, Who loved us and gave us everlasting consolation and encouragement and well-founded hope through [His] grace (unmerited favor), comfort and encourage your hearts and strengthen them—make them steadfast and keep them unswerving—in every good work and word.

2 THESSALONIANS 2:16–17 AMP

FIT TIP #2:

The first truth to know is that God loves you and created you for a special purpose. On index cards, write out five truths from God's Word regarding His love for you. Post them everywhere: in your house, your car, or any place you frequent. Read these verses daily and allow God to renew your mind and begin to heal those wounded places where lies have reigned for so long.

2

MISS FIT

A Compromised Life

I sat down one afternoon with Kim, a chiropractic care patient with whom I had been working for several years. I was often frustrated after our visits. Although she claimed to be a believer in Jesus, she continually found herself in compromising relationships. No matter what the reason was for her visits, our conversations seemed to always drift in that direction. Over and over again she would tell me what a "good" man this one was and how successful he was. Yet a few months would pass, and she would be sitting in my office in tears over another failed relationship. Her reason for this particular visit was a desire to lose weight. I had mentioned to her once when she was complaining about her weight that perhaps I could help, and if she wanted to make some changes, I'd be available.

A petite young woman, Kim seemed to carry extra weight around her stomach, hips, and thighs. She admitted that she had tried a popular herbal weight-loss product, but it made her dizzy, jittery, and irritable. She lost a few pounds but had reached a plateau. She added that she had a really hard time giving up chocolate and was considering becoming a vegetarian. (I wonder how many of my patients don't tell me when they resort to unhealthy ways to lose weight and only come to my office when their attempts fail.)

Kim really wanted to lose this weight. She believed that if she were thin she would attract a nice man. Inside, she knew that a healthy relationship with a godly man was not founded on her physical appearance, but she just couldn't rid her mind of how rejected and lonely she felt when she attended church and seemingly went unnoticed by the eligible single men. She expressed, "They only seem to notice the really thin women." I encouraged her that she was more likely to meet God's choice for her if she would make the commitment to herself and the Lord that she would no longer compromise. I felt so strongly in my heart and knew from my own experience that until we fully commit to the Lord, we can't have His best. The desire for a man, for companionship, and for intimacy was so strong that Kim considered anyone suitable who treated her well and gave her the attention she so desperately wanted. This form of compromise only causes pain and frustration. Scripture tells us of a time in history when God's people also compromised.

> So they came to Jerusalem. Then Jesus went into the temple and began to drive out those who bought and sold in the temple, and over-turned the tables of the moneychangers and the seats of those who sold doves. And He would not allow anyone to carry wares through the tem-ple. Then He taught, saying to them, "Is it not written, 'My house shall be called a house of prayer for all nations'? But you have made it a 'den of thieves' " (Mark 11:15–17).

Certain of Israel's religious leaders had turned God's house into a swap meet, and Jesus was angered as He walked in and saw this unholy exchange taking place in the temple at Jerusalem. This was to be a holy place, not a coven of compromises. The place where prayer was to be the primary activity was now given over to the moneychangers. I shared this story with Kim and related it to addictions. Every addictive agent we employ is a form of compromise. From the most seemingly innocent activity to blatant sin, God will show us if what we are doing is inappropriate. Eating, spending money, exercising, acting promiscu-ously, watching television, or seeking ungodly relationships can all serve as agents and substitutes for the true purpose for our body, which is God's temple. Kim used relationships and food as commodities sold in her temple to make her feel good and give her significance.

"Or do you not know that your body is the temple of the Holy Spirit who is in you, whom you have from God, and you are not your own? For you were bought at a price; therefore glorify God in your body and in your spirit, which are God's" (1 Corinthians 6:19–20). We don't belong to ourselves anymore. What we do with our bodies and what we put into our minds as well as our bodies matters. The more we know of God's tremendous love for us and the more we understand just how marvelous a creation we really are, the more we can appreciate the gift of life by taking care of it the best we know how. Glorifying God in our body and our spirit may manifest itself differently in different people, but the principle remains the same: our body is His temple.

I don't know about you, but frequently I used to try to help God. When we don't really know and trust God, part of our human nature feels if we don't do something, we'll miss out on life. When we doubt He will comfort us in times of despair, we turn to food or some other way to soothe our wounds. When we doubt He will provide for us, we resort to worldly ways to meet our needs. One person may turn to a life of crime, while another will work her fingers to the bone, never to get ahead. When Kim doubted or, for that matter, didn't think God cared about her choice for a mate, she sought to solve her problem through changing her appearance, dieting, and trying to find a suitable partner on her own.

> God is not an evil taskmaster waiting to foil our plans and spoil our fun.

God is not an evil taskmaster waiting to foil our plans and spoil our fun. I believe it grieves Him when we try to meet our needs and fulfill our dreams without consulting Him. He really does know what's best for us. As Jeremiah 29:11 says, "For I know the thoughts that I think toward you, says the Lord, thoughts of peace and not of evil, to give you a future and a hope." God has such good plans if we would but seek Him (v. 13). Most of the time our plans lead to heartache and frustration. It's not always a walk in the park when we fully trust God, but we can have a deep confidence that He can and will work everything out according to His will for our lives. Isn't that what we all really want? True peace that only God can provide? I know I do, and I find that to be a huge motivation for trusting God. It's much safer to trust Him than to trust ourselves. I've learned this lesson the hard way.

In order to mature in our life with Christ, there needs to be a death to our way of doing things and a yielding to God's way. In a sense this death to self-control is analogous to Jesus' turning over the tables in the temple. As He begins to show us those areas where we live in compromise, He also shows us a better way. Little by little the layers of compromise are removed and our true purpose can be made manifest.

Though His discipline may seem tough at times, eventually we see that He is so loving that He daily waits with open arms for us to turn our temple into a house of prayer. Then He can spend time with us, loving us, maturing us, and blessing us. He longs for us to choose to follow His way so we can be free of a life of compromise.

Our relationship with the Lord is not a magic lamp. Though Kim agreed, she was still a bit consumed with meeting a man. She, like so many of us, wanted an immediate answer to her prayers. The path I wanted to lead my precious patient on was the path that would give her peace and contentment as the Lord was molding her and shaping her into what He designed her to be. In the process she would learn healthy eating habits that would produce noticeable physical changes on the outside, but greater changes would occur on the inside. Our motivation for intimacy with the Lord cannot merely be to get our needs met. Likewise, I could not honestly tell Kim that if her priorities were in order she would meet the man of her dreams and lose weight. Though many practice and preach this type of convenient Christianity, it's not based on Scripture, and if it did work, I wouldn't be so sure it was *God* answering that prayer.

The truth is that if we have a truly intimate relationship with the Lord, we are less inclined to care about the other issues. When we are so stressed by the cares of this world that they consume our thoughts, conversations, and plans, Jesus is not the first on our list of those we want to please. Matthew 6:33 shows what our priorities should be in a nutshell: "But seek first the kingdom of God, and His righteousness; and all these things shall be added to you." God isn't telling us not to care about anything, but rather not to be captured by anything that would distract us from His plan for our life.

Kim left my office that day feeling a bit encouraged but also afraid of what was to come. We reviewed her diet, and I gave her some suggestions on how to begin achieving healthy weight loss. I encouraged her to write out her prayers and ask the Lord to begin to turn over those tables where she had compromised.

HEART CHANGES LEAD TO BODY CHANGES

I didn't hear from Kim for a while and began to think she had given up on my suggestions. But in a few months Kim returned to my office with a big smile on her face. She said, "Dr. Little, I expected the earth to open up when I began to pray for the Lord to reveal the areas where I was living in compromise. But it didn't." She jokingly said how she was waiting for a voice from heaven to part the clouds while she was power walking and say to her, "Quit eating chocolate!" But as she wrote out her prayers each morning, she prayed that God would speak to her. Sometimes she would have a thought about an old boyfriend, and in her heart she sensed the need to let it go. These experiences continued to occur over several months, until she knew God had made some pretty huge changes in her heart. She no longer felt the desperation to meet a man. She no longer obsessed about her weight. And most of all, she had a renewed relationship with Jesus. She found that the eating habits were getting easier, and she wasn't experiencing as many ups and downs in her weight. It just wasn't a big deal anymore. What amazed her most was how her attention could now be focused on her work, her devotions, and paying attention in church. Instead of looking around for a good-looking guy when the pastor said, "Please bow your heads," she actually kept her eyes closed and prayed.

The diet changes I suggested to her were based on her cravings. I have found that a person's predominant cravings are a good indication of what type of foods they need to bring about balance. There are two basic categories of cravings: sugars and stimulants, and salts and fats. These cravings tell me which hormone-producing gland is weak and which one is strong. Cravings are a hormonal response to imbalances in the body. We often just think of hormones in regard to "that time of the month." But in actuality, the hormonal—or endocrine—system is one of the most complex of all the body's systems. Hormones control a multitude of functions in our bodies. It is a sensitive network of interrelated chemical-producing glands that work together to keep us healthy. Only slight changes can alter the entire body's hormonal balance.

Everyone's clock ticks in a different way. For one person, a serving of fruit is all she needs for breakfast to have the energy and vitality to get through the morning. Another woman would feel as if her brain were stuffed with cotton if she ate fruit in the morning; she would benefit from eggs and whole-grain toast. Diets are as unique and individual as we are. We can't give everyone the same diet (eating program) and expect to get the same results. Unique people require unique programs. As long as individual nutritional needs are met, there are no good diets or bad diets even though, obviously, there are good foods and bad foods. There is only a right diet for a person based on her individual biochemistry.

God made the grains as well as the fruits and meats for our use. They are all good, but they are not all beneficial for everyone. We are to choose wisely, having dominion over not only the earth but also our own bodies. Food is not to have dominion over us. Psalm 8:6 shows us one example of the authority God has given us: "You put us in charge of everything you made, giving us authority over all things" (NLT). Our first goal is to choose the best quality foods, and then to learn what our individual bodies specifically need. This is a truly freeing experience.

> # As long as individual nutritional needs are met, there are no good diets or bad diets.

We can be freed of media pressure that would have us believe "milk does a body good" when our body may not be able to tolerate milk. Or free not to include XYZ cereal brand as a *part* of our total breakfast, when cereal makes us sleepy and bloated an hour after it's eaten. Notice that cereal is recommended as *part* of a total breakfast, but they neglect to tell you what the other part should be. Since we typically don't pay close attention to commercials, most people miss the little word *part.* Imagine a surgeon telling an anxiously waiting family, "Everything went well; we were able to remove *part* of the tumor." I don't think this would be acceptable. But we accept what we hear when we don't pay attention, and in the case of diet, mindlessly venture off to the market to buy what has been programmed into our minds.

I love how the *New Living Translation* of Psalm 139:14 expresses David's appreciation for the gift of life he was given: "Thank you for making me so wonderfully complex! Your workmanship is marvelous—and how well I know it." As we grow to know, accept, and appreciate our wonderful complexities, we can begin to find freedom from the hold food has on us and move on to being and doing what God has planned.

Kim craved chocolate. Not just sometimes, but all the time. When she was sad, happy, or bored, she'd rather have chocolate than breath. She liked chocolate cake, chocolate candy, chocolate-covered pretzels, and chocolate in her coffee. If it didn't have chocolate on it or in it, she wasn't interested. This fact, coupled with where her body put the extra weight, on her stomach, hips, and thighs, revealed that her adrenal glands were weak and her thyroid was in overdrive. The stimulants kept her motor revved up and in constant "go" mode. The best suggestion for Kim was to eliminate the stimulants. Unfortunately, that meant the chocolate had to go, along with the coffee and the muffins, cookies, pancakes, bagels, sodas, and even great amounts of fruit. The heavens didn't part, but they might as well have. She was not happy about that suggestion.

Simply put, the adrenal glands are our stress-fighting glands. They produce adrenalin, DHEA, cortical-steroids, estrogen, and numerous other chemicals when we go through menopause. When they are weak, we gain weight more easily, retain water, or become more susceptible to colds. The key to bringing Kim's body back into balance was to eliminate those foods that were stressing her body and increase those foods that would strengthen her. The strengthening foods in her case would be fish, eggs, and poultry at every meal, along with her choice of steamed or raw vegetables and a single serving of rice or a whole grain (e.g., oatmeal or bread). The portions were not as significant as long as her meals were balanced throughout the day. The most important factor was to reduce the refined carbohydrates, sugars, and stimulants. After a few days, she would feel her body beginning to stabilize, and the cravings for chocolate would diminish. Eating a small amount of protein every two hours is sometimes a good way to balance the blood sugar. After that, the life plan for maintenance is to eat balanced meals, including animal protein three times per day with no snacking, if possible.

MAKE THE BEST CHOICE POSSIBLE

I told Kim that at every meal she should try to make the best choice possible. Since she had been a specialist in microwave cooking, this took some work. She notoriously would skip breakfast. If she had anything, it would be a cup of coffee on the run. The word *breakfast* implies breaking the fast after a good night's sleep. This means eating in the morning. This charges the batteries and gives the body the energy needed to get through the morning. Since we are all so different, one person's choice for breakfast is not ideal for someone else. The best way to determine if a meal is balanced is to pay attention an hour after eating. If you feel tired or foggy, then the meal was not balanced. The goal is to try different combinations until the perfect balance is achieved. For one person, eggs give that needed morning energy, while another needs something light like fruit and unsalted nuts. Each person is different, but I find the cravings method to be a great place to start. Cravings are different from simply enjoying eating something. Cravings are deep, driving forces that almost speak to you and tell you they want attention, and nothing else seemingly will satisfy.

If Kim had craved potato chips and fried foods instead of chocolate, her diet suggestions would have been completely different. Weight gain would have tended to be on the stomach and back. Salt and fat cravings indicate the adrenal glands are in overdrive and the thyroid and pituitary are the weakened glands. The key here is to eat a diet low in salt, animal protein, and fatty foods and high in fruits, vegetables, and complex carbohydrates. Proteins like chicken, eggs, or fish should be eaten lightly and mostly at dinnertime. Breakfast would consist of a whole-grain cereal or fruit. Lunch would be a big salad with loads of vegetables, broiled fish, and a light olive oil and vinegar dressing with a healthy whole-grain roll and a piece of fruit for dessert. Dinner would include broiled fish or chicken, brown rice or potato, steamed or sautéed vegetables, and a piece of fruit for dessert.

> The word *breakfast* implies breaking the fast after a good night's sleep. This means eating in the morning.

When we make substitutions, we want to substitute for a whole food product. For example, in a low-salt diet, use sea salt and use it sparingly rather than using a low-salt product. The same goes for fats. Rather than use a low-fat salad dressing, use an expeller-pressed olive oil and organic apple cider vinegar with some fresh herb seasoning. Always make the healthier choice.

Kim was considering becoming a vegetarian, thinking that it would be healthier for her. Many respected people in ministry and clinical practice believe humankind is supposed to be vegetarian. I don't agree. Genesis 9:3 tells me, "Every moving thing that lives shall be food for you; and as I gave you the green plants, I give you everything" (RSV). I'm not sure if prior to the flood people ate meat, but my understanding of this verse is that animal products are given to us for food along with vegetables. But what's available today is a bit different than in Noah's day. It's not the product that's bad; it's what has been done to it. If only meats and animal products loaded with chemicals, drugs, hormones, steroids, etc. were available, then I would agree, don't eat animal products. Unfortunately, this goes beyond animal products and into every food God made. People have tried to change every food to make it last longer and look better on the shelf. But, fortunately, most of us in North America do have choices. In most neighborhoods there are sources of produce, meats, and dairy products that are free of adulteration. Choose those before trying to go vegan.

> # Every cell, organ, tissue, and function in our body needs protein.

The fact is that every cell, organ, tissue, and function in our body needs protein. Every cell. Even our hormones are protein in nature. Protein must be picked up daily from our food intake and cannot be stored. Animal protein is the only source that contains all the essential amino acids needed. According to Dr. Louis Rubel, in *The GP and the Endocrine Glands*, "Any tissue of the body deprived of sufficient protein will give rise to symptoms . . . complaints of fatigue, sensitivity to cold, evident pallor, and a negative attitude."[1] He goes on to mention several disorders linked to either protein deficiency or protein mal-digestion: rheumatoid arthritis; diabetes; aches; painful joints; ulcers; colds; tendency to bruise easily; constipation; ankle swelling; brittle nails; dry skin, hair, and eyes; sinusitis; and indigestion.

Include a variety of protein sources in small, frequent portions, including meat, fish, fowl, eggs, cheese, cottage cheese, gelatin, and high-protein cereals. Though I know the people who promote vegetarianism have good intentions, there's simply too much scientific data to support our need for some animal protein. I have a link on my Web site to a site on facts about vegetarianism.

The combination of improving her relationship with the Lord, spending less time looking for a man, and working on her diet has made Kim a happier person. Kim and I spoke weekly for our coaching and praying sessions. Some weeks were awesome and others were total disasters. No matter how many steps were taken forward and how many back, we just kept at it. Success isn't measured by how many good days you have or by how many inches you lose, it is measured by how many times after having fallen down you get back up. Kim's success didn't happen overnight and was not without setbacks, disagreements, and struggles. Slowly, step by step, she was able to let go and trust that this was truly the best plan. She has more energy, enjoys planning her meals, and has started to see this way of eating as a lifestyle and not a weight-loss program. And she no longer has "octopus tentacles" ready to wrap themselves around any unsuspecting single guy.

Perhaps Kim's story hit home for you. You realize that your true motivation for wanting to lose weight is based on a false foundation. Just as God has worked to erect a healthy foundation in Kim's life, He can do the same for you, if you ask Him and trust Him. Let me lead you in a first-step prayer.

Father, I come to you in your Son Jesus' name. I ask you to forgive me for using my temple as a den of thieves, making food my comfort and my weight my gauge. I surrender to you and ask that you would lead me into the right path with a pure heart. Help me to have the right motives for being healthy and losing weight. Help me to be patient with the process and to trust you as you begin to turn over the tables of compromise in my life. Help me to seek first your kingdom and your righteousness and trust you for the rest. I want to find my worth and approval in you and not in food, people, or things. I thank you for loving me. In Jesus' name. Amen.

Beloved, I pray that you may prosper in every way
and [that your body] may keep well, even as [I know]
your soul keeps well and prospers.

3 JOHN 2 AMP

FIT TIP #3:

Let your food cravings tell you what diet is best for you. A craving for sweets, coffee, fruits, and refined carbohydrates indicates a need to increase the protein and cut out the stimulants. A craving for salty and fatty foods indicates a need to increase the fruits, whole grains, low-fat dairy products, and vegetables and go easy on the animal protein.

FIT TIP #4:

Eat breakfast. If your cravings typically are for salty or fatty foods, have some fruit or whole-grain cereal for breakfast. If you crave sugars, pastas, and bread, have eggs cooked in butter or hard-boiled with a slice of whole-grain toast and some turkey sausage.

FIT TIP #5:

As long as nutritional needs are met, there are no good or bad diets—only the right diet for you. Don't allow yourself to be influenced by what the advertisements say is healthy.

FIT TIP #6:

When you blow it, and we all do, don't quit; make a decision to do better at your next meal. Remember, it's not how many times you fall down that counts but how many times you get back up and keep moving.

3
FIT TO BE TIED

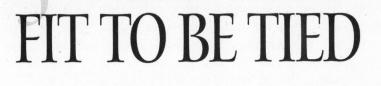

Frustration With Diets and Exercise

Claudia was a woman in her early forties. She had called for an appointment after a good friend from church had suggested her weight frustrations could be nutritional in nature. Since her friend had had success working with me, she thought Claudia might benefit as well. On that first visit, we talked about her frustrations with dieting and exercise. She shared how she couldn't believe that she hadn't lost a pound after working out at the gym every day, taking aerobics for an hour, and running in the evenings. She had cut back her calorie intake to almost nothing but still had not lost one single pound. She admitted that at first, after having her baby, she had been a bit lax with her eating habits because she was just too tired. She had gained forty pounds, but then felt her new self-discipline would cause this extra weight to come off easily. But it hadn't. So Claudia sat in my office angry, teary-eyed, and wondering if anything could be done to help her. She was worn out, "fit to be tied," but not an inch thinner.

I have worked with several other individuals who have had similar frustrations. As we explored Claudia's history, I saw that she had destroyed her metabolism, as many do, through the relentless fad diets she tried after having a baby two years earlier. Her stress level was at a peak, yet she persisted in this insane manner with no results. Her home life suffered because she was so consumed with her weight that she didn't give much attention to her husband or her baby. So much effort and energy expended and nothing in return.

Her husband was supportive and just wanted his wife back. He didn't care if she was heavy or thin; he just wanted her at home more often. Between work and workouts, he was feeling neglected. He had his hobbies, played a little golf, and went fishing every now and then, but really enjoyed being at home with his family. Claudia seemed to have a different agenda. Somehow she had convinced herself that he would leave her if she became overweight. He had never said such a thing, but this didn't change the lies that were in her head. Isn't it amazing how people who love us can tell us over and over how special or beautiful we are and yet we still believe the lie?

I asked Claudia if there had been a time in her life when she felt she would be rejected or left out if she wasn't perfect. She said she would think about it and get back to me. When she did, it was an eye-opening revelation. When she was a child she had been a very talented gymnast. Claudia "knew" that to be any good as a gymnast, she had to be thin and have perfect control over her body. She was diligent and worked at being her best. Her efforts paid off with award after award. Life was starting to present a promising future for Claudia. One afternoon while training, she fell and tore a ligament in her ankle. With a competition just days away, someone else on her team replaced her. Devastated, she was forced to quit gymnastics. She felt like such a failure. She had trained so hard for this competition and now it was all over. She stuffed the pain and blamed herself for the fall. *What a klutz*, she thought. Claudia felt rejected and vowed to never let something like this happen again. That seed of a lie was now in full bloom: If she failed or gained weight, she would not be able to participate in what she enjoyed.

Claudia's story reminds me of the people the prophet Haggai spoke about in the Old Testament:

> "Is it time for you yourselves to dwell in your paneled houses, and this temple to lie in ruins?" Now therefore, thus says the Lord of hosts:
> "Consider your ways!
> You have sown much, and bring in little;

You eat, but do not have enough;
You drink, but you are not filled with drink;
You clothe yourselves, but no one is warm;
And he who earns wages,
Earns wages to put into a bag with holes" (Haggai 1:4–6).

They were so consumed with their paneled houses that the temple was in ruins. They were also frustrated since all of their efforts seemed to be thwarted without reward. But they, like Claudia, kept doing the same things over and over with no positive results. Have you ever watched a fly on a window? An open door may be just two feet away, but the fly will try incessantly to get through the closed window until finally the buzzing tones down, it quits, and dies. A solution is sometimes so close, but we can't see it because we are consumed with our own fruitless solutions.

God gave these frustrated, superficial people a message through the prophet Haggai and strongly encouraged them to stop and think about what they were doing. Sometimes we, too, need to stop and consider our ways.

What was Claudia willing to risk to have the perfect body? Fortunately she was unsuccessful at her way of achieving her goals. Otherwise, she might have lost her life, her family, or at the least destroyed her health. I believe God would tell Claudia to consider her ways as well.

> ## What was Claudia willing to risk to have the perfect body?

God showed His people that the solution was to return to the basics and do first things first. "Thus says the Lord of hosts: 'Consider your ways! Go up to the mountains and bring wood and build the temple, that I may take pleasure in it and be glorified,' says the Lord" (Haggai 1:7–8).

Whatever our endeavor, if God isn't glorified, it isn't worth our effort. Scripture goes on to tell us that even when these people thought they had succeeded, God thwarted their plans. But they finally obeyed the Lord's command and did as He said. He didn't leave them buzzing against a closed window; He opened a door for them that was better than before.

I performed an evaluation on Claudia and she left my office with a diet diary in hand. I encouraged her that God would give her strength as we pursued the truth of her health issues. Thread by thread we would work to untie the knots in her life and lead her to freedom.

EMPTY NUTRIENTS LEAD TO VIRTUAL STARVATION

On Claudia's return visit, we were armed and ready to begin loosening the ties that had her so firmly bound. The examination had revealed vitamin, mineral, and digestive enzyme deficiencies. As we looked through her diet diary, there was more white space than ink. She was consumed with eating empty-nutrient, low-calorie, and low-fat foods. She had lived this way for so long that she was rarely hungry. She thought this was good, since the less she ate, the better chance she had of losing the weight. But she was starving her body. As she began to understand, she realized that this virtual starvation explained her extreme fatigue and continual feeling of being bloated. If she were a car, the engine would have burned up for lack of oil.

> If she were a car, the engine would have burned up for lack of oil.

The first step in her healing process was to replenish the nutrients she had lost and replenish the digestive enzymes she needed to properly digest food. Our nutritional needs vary, so I don't recommend everyone take vitamins and minerals. But in Claudia's case, we needed to primarily replenish potassium and zinc. I gave her an organic multiple vitamin and an organic mineral supplement.[1] I was very specific in what I recommended. Only what we found to be deficient was given and no more.

Next, we dealt with her dietary changes. She was instructed to eat five small "protein" meals per day. This was to be done for one month, and then she could reduce her meals to three per day. By this time her body would be stronger and her blood sugar more stable. I suggested protein foods such as eggs, fish, chicken, unsalted raw nuts, and cottage cheese. At each meal she would have some protein along with either a vegetable or piece of fruit as well as a healthy fat. Healthy fats include butter, olive oil, flaxseed oil, and any expeller-pressed oil.

I know combining fruit, starch, fats, and proteins raises the hair on the back of the necks of those who support combining only certain foods, but I do not find clinical evidence to support their theory. I believe we are fearfully and wonderfully made, and our bodies have the ability to discern in a meal what is a carbohydrate and what is a protein. For those of you unaware of the food combining theories, some believe that foods of certain types should not be eaten together, such as fruit and protein. Nevertheless, it has been my clinical experience that only those critically ill benefit from particular food combining, because their digestive systems are so fragile.

I gave Claudia a hunger scale to follow. The hunger scale is a way to gain control over your appetite and to become more aware of how your body recognizes hunger and fullness. I asked her to become aware of the ranges of her hunger during the day. On a scale of one to four, with one representing starvation and four stuffed, she was to begin eating at a two and stop at a three. As she continued to journal her eating, she also would journal her feelings. This would help her tap into how certain foods made her feel and how her hunger changed based on the stress in her life. Awareness of the role her emotions played in her appetite helped her to see areas where she needed to focus more attention in her prayer time.

Little by little, her energy returned, and she slowly began to lose weight. The process didn't occur overnight. Her deficiencies had seriously compromised her health. Before her body would let go of extra weight, it needed to be confident it was going to receive the nutrition it had lost. It took more than eleven months for her to take off the forty pounds. But as she shifted her priorities back onto the Lord and His path to a fulfilling life, she began to sense that her life could and would be restored. She wasn't only physically run down; she was spiritually run down as well. She rarely spent time in prayer—except for an occasional pocket prayer for a parking space or to lessen the traffic. She hadn't picked up her Bible in so long it was blending in with the scenery on her bedroom dresser.

When Claudia slowed down enough to see how her life really looked, she saw such emptiness that she wondered how she had survived this long. She realized that it would take much time alone with God to restore what had been lost. I suggested that she take "walks with God" each morning. Instead of focusing on how many calories she could burn, she was to focus on her heavenly Father. As she walked, listening to praise and worship music, she learned to adore her Father, and eventually she rediscovered who she really was. Her walks with God became so enjoyable that sometimes she would not walk at all, but sit in the park watching the children play. Her appreciation for life grew, as did her love for her family. She no longer resented the beautiful little girl that God had given her, blaming the child for her weight gain. God had blessed her, but she had been too busy to see it.

BELIEVING THE LIE

Next, we focused on the lies she believed. In her journal, Claudia began to write down the false beliefs she had accumulated. She started with the lie that if she gained weight her husband would leave her. I suggested that we first focus on God's truth, and then on the facts. Truths like "I will never leave you nor forsake you" (Hebrews 13:5) and "While we were still sinners, Christ died for us" (Romans 5:8) to show that God loved her, imperfections and all. Even when we fail, our heavenly Father is faithful and promises never to let us go.

After focusing on the truth of God's Word, Claudia could turn her focus to the facts. Her husband had proven character; he was a godly man. He had shown her that he had integrity. Not that he was perfect, but she knew he was an honest man. She needed to believe him, only second to believing God. If she was going to remain married to this man, she needed to deal with her fears and believe him when he said he loved her and didn't care how much she weighed. When the lies would slam her, she was now equipped with the armor of the Word of God to punch back with true power. She wrote the Scriptures on cards and posted them everywhere until she had them memorized. After a while, she was able to relax and not allow her fears to drive her. We all know the Enemy doesn't give up, but as she applied this technique to new false statements that came to mind, she found victory.

Excessive exercise can cause more harm than good.

Last, I suggested she stop working out at the gym for a while. Her body needed a break. She had been overdoing it. Her workouts were stressful to her body, and at this point not helpful. They were actually hindering her from losing weight and being healthy. Her walks in the morning would be sufficient to keep her toned and give her the boost she needed. She would be able to return to the gym when her body was stronger and her immune system healthier. It is hard to imagine that excessive exercise can cause more harm than good, but it does and more often than I'd like to admit. Many well-intentioned people are destroying their health by working out more than is healthy. The key is balance. If you've been overdoing it, give it a rest for a while and start back with a game plan that is balanced and healthy. Great results can be achieved by exercising twenty minutes per day or a more strenuous workout only three days per week.

Does Claudia remind you of anyone? Maybe she's a reflection of you. Do you find that no matter how hard you try to lose weight, your efforts are frustrated? Your family—or maybe your work—is neglected. You realize something needs to change. Have you believed some of the lies that the Enemy throws at you? If yes, then pray with me.

Father, I come to you in spirit and in truth. Your Word is a lamp unto my feet and a light unto my path. Reveal yourself through your Word and show me the ways that are unpleasing to you. Reveal the lies of the Enemy that I have believed and that have kept me bound and unable to walk in the freedom you have so freely given me. Forgive me for believing those lies and help me to believe the truth. Where my efforts have been futile, give me comfort and peace as I turn my plans and heart's desires over to you. For I want your will to be done in my life: weight, family, home, and work. I yield to you, Lord God, for your way is perfect. In Jesus' name. Amen.

And we know that all things work together for good to those who love God, to those who are the called according to His purpose.

ROMANS 8:28

FIT TIP #7:

Follow the hunger scale with every meal. On a scale of one to four, one is being starved and four is feeling stuffed. Begin eating at two and stop at three. This will help minimize the triggers to overeat due to being starved and will minimize the digestive discomfort that results from overeating.

FIT TIP #8:

Take walks with God. Instead of being focused on yourself and your weight, let each day be an opportunity to pray for those you love, your neighbors, your city, or the nation. At the end of each walk, journal your thoughts and observations and watch what God will do.

FIT TIP #9:

Don't ignore your emotions and thoughts. Instead, put them to the test. If the feeling or thought is not based on God's truth as revealed in His Word, then find a Scripture to replace the lie. Write it on several cards and place them all over your house, car, and day planner. Anywhere you will see it, post it. Memorize the verses, and when the lie comes into your head, focus on the truth you know, and that truth will set you free.

FIT TIP #10:

Exercise in moderation. Some people benefit most from a brisk walk, while others like the exhilaration of a run on a path or on the beach. Weight training is an excellent way to tone and build muscle. Each person's body has different requirements. Listen to your body, and don't ignore the warning signals. Don't exercise if you are weak and tired. As you pay attention to your body's signals, tailor a workout that suits you best.

4
TWENTY-FOUR-HOUR FITNESS

Holding Onto a Goal

I bumped into Melissa at the market. She had the look of a child who'd just been caught doing something naughty. I hate feeling like the diet police. She had cancelled her appointment again, and I was curious as to what was going on. Without my saying anything, as if she knew what I was going to say, she spewed out a mile-long list of reasons why she had cancelled her appointment and how the timing wasn't right. After talking for a while, we agreed on a meeting the next day to discuss what was really going on and come up with a new strategy to help her reach and maintain her goal.

On her last visit, I had thought she was finally ready to make the leap. She had been putting off her appointment for months, but finally was so disgusted that she called my office. She admitted to being frustrated with not being able to wear her "cute" clothes, and as she put it, "I'll do anything to get this weight off. I feel so ugly." I'll admit, I get excited when a patient is truly committed to changing. I'll do anything to support someone who is doing his or her best to accomplish specific health and weight-loss goals. Sometimes I think I want to see a patient reach her goal more than she does, and I get really upset when she quits prior to reaching it. I know both personally and clinically how satisfying it is to reach a goal. But the process may seem so far off that many people can't imagine it or can't hold onto the vision long enough to reach their destination. Apparently that had been true of Melissa.

Over the next few months I learned that Melissa based many of her decisions on how she felt at that particular moment. If she felt ugly and fat, she wanted a diet. But when she felt depressed, she wanted to pacify the pain with brownies. The diet got thrown out the window, and the emotion of the moment was satisfied. Her diet was controlled by her feelings, and this, unfortunately, was a reflection of her entire life. As I climbed onto this roller coaster with Melissa, I realized what a destructive way of living this was, and I needed to be careful.

A classic extrovert, Melissa was bubbly, fun, and seemed to know everyone in town. Her work brought her in front of many people, and she loved that. People energized her. She had a tough time being alone. But when she was in a crowd, mingling with the local who's who, she was in her element. She walked fast, talked fast, and made decisions fast. Her impulsiveness was great for her work but not for her health. She grew up in a large family, the youngest child and everyone's darling. Love was given freely and abundantly. She learned from a very young age what would get her what she wanted. If she wanted her big brother to give her a ride, she put on a pouty face; he'd melt and do anything for her. Basically she was spoiled rotten and never required to grow up. In a sense, Melissa was emotionally a four-year-old child. Old enough to make some decisions but not to fully understand the consequences.

> Every program works to some degree. So why are more people fighting obesity than ever in the history of our country?

Ask anyone; I don't mind spoiling my patients. Everyone needs to be shown extra love, but there comes a point when I realize that may not serve the patient's overall best interest. Some people want me to do all the work for them. Melissa was committed to the idea of losing weight but not to the process. She would get excited during our appointments and assure me that she would follow through. But then, sure enough, when the diet didn't feel right anymore or she couldn't manage her cravings, she would quit. I needed to learn some new skills as a clinician in order to help this very vivacious young woman reach the goals she really wanted.

It's assumed in most conventional therapies that all that is needed is a desire to change and a good, solid program, and excellent results will follow. But what I have come to see over the past several years is that the program is almost last in significance. Every program works to some degree. So why are more people fighting obesity than ever in the history of our country? I believe it is because most effective programs start with the assumption that everyone who says she wants to lose weight is ready to make permanent and immediate lifestyle changes.

Of course, we are inundated with programs that offer short-term immediate success with little or no lifestyle changes required. Thousands of people are fooled every day into thinking that the weight they lose on one of these programs will be permanent. But for those who seek a legitimate weight-loss program, most of the programs available start out with the common assumption that the person is really ready to change. The results prove this untrue. Different people are in different stages of readiness and require different levels and degrees of support. If Melissa—and many good-intentioned people who base their reality on how they feel—didn't drop a reasonable amount of weight in the first week, she would get depressed and quit. In a sense, she gave me a one-week window of opportunity to get her so motivated that she would hang in there. Since this was both unhealthy and ineffective in the long run, I needed new strategies to help her.

If Melissa had had her way, I would have become an appendage, following her around twenty-four hours a day like a guardian angel. Sitting on her shoulder, I would be her constant reminder and instructor. *Time to snack, Melissa; time to take your supplements, Melissa; time to eat lunch, Melissa; don't eat that roll, Melissa; choose the water instead of the soda, Melissa. . . .* She really did not want to do the work to reach her goal. But this wasn't realistic. Responsibility is needed if we are going to mature and grow and become all we are destined to be. I wondered if something traumatic was going to have to happen in order for her to "get it." For many, this is what's necessary. In many twelve-step programs, this place is called *rock bottom*. Some of us need to hit rock bottom before we can look up and see how foolish we've been. I hoped I could reach Melissa before she reached rock bottom. God doesn't cause the bottom to drop out in our lives, but He doesn't always stop it from happening, especially if that is what will ultimately draw us closer to Him and transform us into the image of Jesus.

THE ROOT ISSUES

After running several tests, we found the chemical root to Melissa's weight challenges, but more than the chemical imbalances, we also needed to address another root issue: Melissa was totally submitted to the wrong god—her feelings. This may not seem dangerous on the surface, but it is. God wants His children to be controlled by His Spirit. If our flesh is in control, we are out of alignment and a target for the Enemy. Anything can throw off our good intentions if we're not fully submitted to God. More important, this attitude was one of pride for Melissa, and unfortunately, it permeates our society, even in the church. What seemed like an innocent woman not willing to take responsibility for her actions was really pride cloaked in irresponsibility.

Melissa did not want to take responsibility for her life and until this point didn't realize it. She just thought she was too busy to put a concerted effort toward her own health and well-being. The right timing is also what the man was waiting for at the pool in Bethesda. When the angel stirred the water, he waited for someone to come along and put him in the pool. Day in and day out he would miss his opportunity at wholeness because he waited, because he did not take responsibility for his own health.

> Now there is in Jerusalem by the Sheep Gate a pool, which is called in Hebrew, Bethesda, having five porches. In these lay a great multitude of sick people, blind, lame, paralyzed, waiting for the moving of the water. For an angel went down at a certain time into the pool and stirred up the water; then whoever stepped in first, after the stirring of the water, was made well of whatever disease he had.
>
> Now a certain man was there who had an infirmity thirty-eight years. When Jesus saw him lying there, and knew that he already had been in that condition a long time, He said to him, "Do you want to be made well?"
>
> The sick man answered Him, "Sir, I have no man to put me into the pool when the water is stirred up; but while I am coming, another steps down before me."
>
> Jesus said to him, "Rise, take up your bed and walk."
>
> And immediately the man was made well, took up his bed, and walked. (John 5:2–9)

Excuses, excuses! Jesus did not ask him if he needed help getting into the pool. He simply asked him *if* he wanted to be made well. This man's issue was not what to do but if he really wanted the result he had been waiting to receive for thirty-eight years. He had come to accept that unless someone else did the work for him, nothing would change. His focus was on getting help to get into the water rather than on getting well or on who could make him well.

Melissa said she wanted to lose weight and complained incessantly about it, but had not yet truly made up her mind that she would do what she needed to do to reach her goal. I suggested to her that she write down the ten reasons why she did not want to lose weight. After she argued that she *did* want to, I showed her that her actions spoke louder than her words.

Our next step was to create some short-term goals with big rewards that she could easily implement. We accomplished this through weekly coaching sessions. Her first assignment was the hardest. She was to do

Create some short-term goals with big rewards.

something she had never done in her life: write out a grocery list with all the healthy foods she enjoyed and that were good for her. She also needed to throw out and refuse to buy again all the foods that were triggers for her. She would no longer keep potato chips and ice cream in the house and no longer buy cookies. Instead, she stocked her fridge with fresh vegetables, unsalted raw nuts, and even some healthy protein bars. She wasn't much interested in cooking, but I convinced her to eat breakfast at home and take healthy snacks to work. She could still go out to dinner often, but she knew her danger zones and strictly avoided them. She made a list of the restaurants that offered a nice selection of foods that were on her healthy food list and began to initiate asking her friends to dinner at her safe-zone spots.

When we talked each week, she would share her successes and struggles with me. She came up with a list of rewards that were not food based. For example, to get a massage, facial, or manicure and pedicure, or to walk on the beach at sunset with a close friend were some of her rewards. If she spent the week staying focused on her goal, she got the reward. Melissa was so affected by her environment that the concept of safe zones was helpful to her. At work, at home, in her car, and even socially, she made sure she was surrounded by people, places, and things that were in line with her new commitment to reaching her goals.

She even had a few friends that she could not hang out with until she was stronger both in her faith and in her diet. Whenever she went out with this select few, she would blow it. She spoke with them about her goals and asked if they would be supportive, but once they went out she saw that they weren't helping her. So for a season she let these relationships go.

Next, we needed to focus on the words that came out of her mouth. I wanted her to stop saying that she was ugly when she was heavier than she wanted to be. Whether she was physically striking or not, she was still beautiful. This was now one of her goals: to find and meditate on what the Scriptures say about true beauty. It's definitely healthier if our words and beliefs about ourselves are consistent with what God says. I have observed that as our words and our intentions become more congruent, the actions that follow flow out of truth and not fear or some other unhealthy emotion.

As Melissa became more consistent with her eating habits and more aware of her triggers, as well as how to readily access the tools she was now armed with, she began to lose weight. She was healthy, and there was really no reason she should have extra weight on her body. She just had some really bad habits and an altar erected to the god of the senses.

METABOLIC EVALUATION

When I evaluate a patient, I ask certain questions regarding what foods she likes or craves, what she eats for breakfast, at what times during the day she feels most tired, how many hours of sleep she gets per night, and so on. The answers clue me in to what is occurring metabolically. Melissa complained of allergies that seemed to be seasonal, and she noticed she had been getting colds more frequently. Worst of all, she felt "puffy" all the time. One day she could wake up, get on the scale, and seem to have gained five pounds overnight. She also noticed her muscles weren't as toned as they used to be. She jokingly frowned as she wiggled the loose flesh on the back of her arms, saying that her arms looked like a turkey's neck. Her weight gain was mostly around her waist and upper body. "What does this all mean, Dr. Little?" she asked with exasperation.

A simple in-office urinary adrenal function test confirmed that Melissa was dealing with adrenal stress. This would explain her fatigue and weight gain that was really fluid retention in disguise. In other words, Melissa's immune system was "wiped out." This is caused by prolonged mental or emotional, chemical or nutritional, physical or electromagnetic (excessive cellular phone use) stress, leading the adrenal glands to decrease their production of cortisol and adrenaline. A healthy response to stress would be a temporary increase in cortisol and adrenaline. With chronic stress, the body eventually hits the wall, and forces the cortisol and adrenaline to decrease in production.

Many people don't understand how significant stress is or, for that matter, *what* stress is. It is one of the main risk factors in disease that can be controlled, but it must first be understood. Melissa commented when I broached the subject of stress that she didn't "feel" stressed. But stress is not something we necessarily feel; it is how our bodies respond to life. The world-renowned researcher on stress, Dr. Hans Selye, defines stress in his classic book *The Stress of Life* as "the rate of wear and tear in the body. The word *stress*, in this sense, designates the sum of all the nonspecific effects of factors (normal activity, disease-producers, drugs, etc.) which can act upon the body."[1]

If the activities of our lives, our genetic inheritance, our diets, and our emotional management are all in balance and order, our response to any excessive load will be one of resilience and not disease. But if our system is out of balance, we will not be

> ## Stress is not something we necessarily feel; it is how our bodies respond to life.

able to maintain balance under the impact of stressors, and we will sooner or later manifest disease. According to Dr. Selye, there are three stages to the stress response. The first is the alarm stage, in which our bodies are responding to an emergency or trauma. This phase should not last long, and adaptation, or stage two, should occur, returning the body back to balance, stage three, within a short amount of time. If the stressor persists, or if the person has destroyed this mechanism through poor diet and emotional management skills, the body will not adapt and return to balance but will stay in the alarm mode until it is exhausted. Unfortunately for many people, life is just plain exhausting. The on-the-go-with-too-much-to-do lifestyle keeps the body in alarm mode. For Melissa, her body had been in a constant state of alert for so long it was now exhausted. She used to be so energetic; now she was always tired but still maintained the same schedule and pseudo-energetic façade that she felt was needed to remain "socially acceptable."

Prolonged stress and her always-needing-to-be-on-the-go attitude were slowly ruining Melissa's immune system. Much of her weight problem was really due to stress. The solution was first to convince Melissa that her to-do list did not need to be filled each day. Just because there were twenty-five spaces on her day planner page didn't mean she had to complete twenty-five tasks.

I placed Melissa on a whole-food-based mineral that contained magnesium and potassium to alleviate the stress on her adrenals, causing her to lose minerals through the urine and stress her kidneys, and I gave her an herbal combination that contained licorice, turmeric, gotu kola, and black currant. I also recommended a B$_6$-Niacinimide supplement.[2] The primary issue in strengthening her adrenals was to eliminate all stimulants, such as sugar, caffeine, fructose, and even any natural remedies that would further tax her already stressed immune system. Though this meant no more mocha lattes in the morning with the gang, she chose the herbal tea and eventually was okay with this choice.

These nutrients, combined with Melissa's new eating habits, were a drastic change from her previous lifestyle. But she knew this was a lifestyle change and not just a "Band-Aid" to get her to feel better and lose weight. Our goal together was to create an entirely new paradigm of planning, stress and emotional management, healthy rewards, and life-regenerating healthy foods. Today Melissa doesn't always make the right choice, but who *always* does the right thing? The main point is that she understands her vulnerable areas and has effective tools to work through them. She has lost the weight and tries to make the choices every day to (1) trust God; (2) obey Him; (3) choose life; and (4) choose balance according to God's will: "Oh, that you would choose life, that you and your descendants might live! Choose to love the Lord your God and to obey him and commit yourself to him, for he is your life. Then you will live long in the land the Lord swore to give your ancestors Abraham, Isaac, and Jacob" (Deuteronomy 30:19–20 NLT).

Although Melissa still loves being the social butterfly, she understands that unless she has balance, she will build disease. This encourages her to take those thoughts captive and to be more aware of her feelings. They don't control her as much now, but she still needs to be on guard when the Enemy gets sneaky and tries to pull a fast one on her.

So many women—and maybe you are one of them—feel that they are completely at the whim of the emotion dominating on any particular day. I believe God has available for you freedom that goes beyond what you eat. His freedom speaks to your core, your heart, to *you*. So many times, out of frustration, we eat to pacify the anxiety within us. If you can relate to Melissa, then pray with me.

> *Father, you knew me before you knit me in my mother's womb. You*
> *know my fears, my anxieties, and my frustrations. I so want to live a*
> *healthy, balanced life. I offer my life to you as a living sacrifice. Take my*
> *life, Lord, and pull up all the holds the Enemy has had on my emotions.*

Draw me closer to you when I feel depressed or afraid of my challenges. I want to have that fruitful, power-filled life that will glorify you. Help me to choose on a moment-by-moment basis to trust you, obey you, and choose to receive your best for me instead of what I may feel is best at the moment. In Jesus' name. Amen.

Trust in the Lord with all your heart; do not depend on your own understanding. Seek his will in all you do, and he will direct your paths.

PROVERBS 3:5–6 NLT

FIT TIP #11:

Be prepared. Never leave home without a plan for your meals for the day. As you plan your week, also plan your meals and snacks. If you know you have meetings or parties scheduled, plan around them so that you are never caught hungry and off guard out in the fast-food wilderness.

FIT TIP #12:

Don't buy any unhealthy snack foods. Keep your environment safe, healthy, and pure. Trust me, if it's in the house, you will eat it.

FIT TIP #13:

Make a list of restaurants that have foods on their menus that you enjoy and that are also healthy for you. When friends ask you out to lunch, ask them if they'd like to try someplace new.

5

FIT FANTASIES

Keys to Unlocking the Prison of Obesity

Julia brought in some old photos of herself to give me an idea of how she used to look. She thought this would be helpful because she had gained more than one hundred pounds over the last ten years. She didn't look like the same person anymore, and I almost found it hard to believe she was. Julia held on to those old photos as she would a long-lost friend.

As I looked at each picture, I saw something in her eyes, the position of her head, the way she held her mouth. It spoke of something beyond trying to look pretty. It was a seductive look. She looked beautiful, but her eyes spoke of lost virtue. It was hard to pinpoint what I saw without more knowledge, but her eyes and body language spoke of something mysterious and dark. I didn't think I was imagining this, but I couldn't draw any conclusions until I knew more about the woman who sat in front of me, hoping I held the keys to unlock her prison of obesity.

Julia had just celebrated her forty-third birthday. Actually this was her motivation to schedule her appointment with me. She had received a gift certificate from her Bible study group to see a nutritionist. Week after week she would ask for prayer that God would help her lose weight. So this was the perfect birthday gift.

Julia was a closet eater. When she was out with her friends she ate very little, but when she was alone she would eat bags of chips, breads, and cheeses. These were her weaknesses. To her, these foods were God's gift to humankind. She loved chips and dip, especially nachos with lots of guacamole, melted cheese, and salsa. She would make nachos at home because she could eat so many it was embarrassing to order them with friends. If she went to a restaurant alone, she ordered whatever she wanted, but she would take at least half of it home in a doggy bag only to finish it off before bedtime. Over several years, this kind of behavior adds up—in pounds as well as in habits. It's really quite simple to lose weight, but breaking bad habits is hard.

Julia's family had lived all over the world. She was the only daughter of a retired navy captain, and she had one brother. Her family moved frequently, as is common in the military. Julia said her mom was a petite, almost boyish-looking woman with a

> It's really quite simple to lose weight, but breaking bad habits is hard.

quiet and unassuming personality. She dressed conservatively and was very proper. As far back as Julia could remember, her mom pretty much maintained the same size.

Julia matured at an early age. She got her first bra at nine and started her period at ten. At the same time, Julia found herself very curious about her sexuality and that of the neighborhood boys, as she would "play doctor" with them. Though she never wanted to draw any attention to herself outside of sports or academic pursuits, she was drawn to entertain her physical passions and curiosities.

Julia recalled when she was a little girl how her mom taught her proper etiquette and how to "be a lady." Julia was encouraged by her mother to accentuate her positive attributes with the use of makeup and more feminine clothing. Since Julia saw herself as a tomboy, she resisted dressing femininely and preferred jeans, a T-shirt, and sneakers. Makeup didn't touch her face until she was in college. Eventually she enjoyed putting on makeup and even dressing more femininely, but deep inside she still felt like a tomboy. She attracted boys from a very young age but never really thought of herself as pretty. When people would tell her she was pretty, she would say thanks in disbelief.

When Julia came to me, she had been seeing a Christian psychologist for quite some time. She would pray with Julia and sought to uncover the root of her challenges from a spiritual perspective. This particular therapist was trained in what many call deliverance prayer or listening prayer in addition to her professional training. Strategically, through the therapist, God uncovered what had been dormant for many years and broke the bars that the Enemy used to keep Julia captive most of her adult life.

There are very few of us who have come to where we are without some form of rejection, abuse, fear, or wounding. If not healed, we wear these wounds like sunglasses, altering our perspective on the world. It's hard to imagine being zealous about spreading the Gospel when we are petrified of what people think of us. It was after addressing long-standing issues that Julia was ready to see me. She shared her experiences with me and some of the things God had shown her through prayer and counseling. She was able to recall some very significant events from her childhood.

Julia remembered the closed door as her parents shared intimate times. But she also remembered going into their bedroom when they were away and looking through their dresser drawers. There she uncovered magazines that were never on the coffee table. They contained pornographic images, which spoiled the innocence of this young, impressionable girl. They frightened her, confused her. Was this what Mom and Dad did behind closed doors? Was this what women did? Was this what she was expected to do? At age seven, all she felt was confused and ashamed. She couldn't ask her mom or dad about it, because she feared they would get angry if they knew she had gone through their things. So she held it inside, only to have the shame and the images remain locked in her soul for years.

As she got older, she began to explore her sexuality, not knowing why or what she was doing. She just felt compelled to do so. Perhaps she was subconsciously living out what was embedded in the foundation of her soul. The damage was leaking out from the cracks of a wounded vessel. She frequently indulged in alcohol and smoked marijuana. She got a kick out of secretly getting high. It was her private party. While still in her teens, she became sexually promiscuous. After all, this was what women did, right? Her promiscuous behavior was very secretive. She would think to herself, *This isn't me. I'm not really like this.* She never told her friends of her secret life. The men she was with were mostly strangers whom she didn't love. A fun-loving young woman, she found it very easy to meet men at the gym or at bars.

Just out of college, after several years of living a double life, one evening Julia went out with a man she had recently met. They ended up at his apartment after dinner, had a few drinks, and then had sex. She was taking the Pill, but had been having problems because the dosage was causing break-through bleeding. He jokingly asked her if she had any diseases. She told him she didn't. But he did. He left her with gonorrhea—and pregnant. The secret would soon be known unless she did something about it. She had her career and future to think about. She wasn't about to become part of the statistics of unwed mothers. She was too young. She didn't love the young man, and besides, he was long gone. She couldn't afford to raise a child. These and hundreds of other reasons why a baby was inconvenient came to her mind. The only option in her thinking was to terminate the pregnancy.

Julia was numb. She felt neither sadness nor pain. Her conscience was seared, and she was past feeling. Somewhere inside of her soul she knew abortion was murder, but her reputation was more important and the fear of being exposed was too great. No one in her family and none of her friends knew of her other life. A baby would definitely merge the two and so had to go. The "procedure" was relatively quick and painless. No different from any other outpatient surgery. The day came and went just like any other day.

We hear of the negative effects of pornography on families and on women, but usually the users are men. Seldom do we hear of the negative impact pornography has on children, especially female children. When Julia first laid eyes on those sexual images, the gate into her soul was invaded. The shame she felt caused her to hide. She continued to sneak peeks into her dad's private stash through her teens. But then the hiding became the rule rather than the exception. Secrets, lies, justification, and hiding were the behaviors that came from her being ashamed.

Those images did not teach Julia what was normal, that sex was a gift from God Almighty, an expression of love to be shared by two people united in marriage. They taught her that it was simply self-gratification at the expense of others. It trivialized that which is sacred and created bonds with fantasy images. It taught her that the woman's role was to please the man at the expense of her dignity. It taught her that *no* was not in the vocabulary. Through pornography, the devil stole Julia's virtue, her *no*, and wiped out any level of self-esteem she had been taught by her parents. Her view of women had been reduced to voiceless objects that needed to look good and perform, and her view of men was a faceless phallic symbol that had needs to be met by the woman. She didn't view men and women as God's beautiful creation, created in His image.

We must not be ignorant of the Enemy's devices to destroy our children. He has been doing this since the beginning of time when he convinced the people to sacrifice their babies to the god of Molech. Ezekiel 16:20–21 conveys the broken heart of God as His children bow to worthless idols. "Moreover, you have taken your sons and your daughters whom you have borne to Me, and you have sacrificed them [to your idols] to be destroyed. Were your harlotries too little, that you have slain My children, and delivered them up, in setting them apart and causing them to pass through the fire for [your idols]?" (AMP). The Enemy is no different today and is still targeting our children through abortion and other vile forms of abuse. Scripture tells us that it is better to have a stone tied around your neck and be cast into the sea than to harm a little child. Matthew 18:6 says, "But whoever causes one of these little ones who believe in Me to sin, it would be better for him if a millstone were hung around his neck, and he were drowned in the depth of the sea." I wonder how many parents don't even realize how they have allowed their own children to be violated by the careless presence of pornographic materials in their home.

GOD WILL SET THE CAPTIVE FREE

No matter how huge the lie of the Enemy, God is able to set the captive free—permanently. It wasn't until Julia's heart was ready that God could reveal the roots of her emotional and physical challenges. Her counseling, the healing prayer, and her own personal time with God brought clarity and wholeness to a picture that had many holes in it. But John 8:32 tells us that we will know the truth and that truth will set us free. The truth to know is that no matter how dark, how awful, how wounded we have been, God loves us. And nothing can or ever will separate us from His love. Just as His love is unconditional, His forgiveness is available to anyone who calls on Him, willing to yield every aspect of her life over to the living God. For this reason Jesus Christ came, to bring good news to the captives, to bind up the brokenhearted, to free the prisoners, and most of all to reconcile us back to our heavenly Father. It was the power of God through prayer and specifically addressing the root cause of Julia's infirmity that brought her out of darkness. It is the power of God that set her free from the bondage of pornography and its related sins of promiscuity and murder.

Little was Julia aware that for years after she terminated her pregnancy, she filled the suppressed guilt from the abortion with activities. Eventually food became her greatest comfort. She no longer wanted to be attractive to men. She began to hate men as well as to hate her own body. She found that certain foods gave her a sense of satisfaction, the richer the better. Cheese, dips, chips, and cheesecakes became her friends. Instead of talking with someone, she held the pain inside, worked hard, and in time gained over one hundred pounds. Dr. Theresa Burke validates this as a common experience among women after having an abortion. She says, "Compulsive overeating may provide momentary comfort and nurturing. People can use eating as a way to calm and soothe anxiety, tension, and emotional pain. It can also become a nervous compulsion that provides a gateway to protective defenses. Overeating may satisfy an unconscious desire to isolate oneself from the source of trauma. After a painful abortion, a woman may try to disconnect from the sexual appeal of a beautiful body. Extra weight can provide a sense of protection from the risk of emotional intimacy."[1] This was true for Julia as it is for many women.

One summer Julia's brother, whom she hadn't seen in years, came to visit her. When she picked him up from the airport, he hardly recognized her. They had a chance to talk, and to her amazement, he had given his life to Jesus Christ and had been

> # Cheese, dips, chips, and cheesecakes became her friends.

faithfully serving Him for many years. He sensed she had an eating problem, and before he left shared with her God's plan for healing a wounded soul and suggested she get some counseling. He bought her a Bible and shared with her some Scriptures relating to God's truth, freedom, and strength.

It was after he left that Julia sought out the psychologist to help her deal with the imbalances in her life. This therapist just "happened" to be a Christian. She spoke to Julia about the love of God as her Father. As a Father, He would love her, protect and provide for her. He would never leave her, and most of all, He would show her through His Word what true fulfillment and love really is. The therapist showed her how the Father sent His only Son, Jesus Christ, as the true expression of love, and that through this love, captives are set free.

Julia had what she thought was a healthy relationship with her dad, but soon was able to see that since her dad didn't know God as his heavenly Father, he had allowed things into their home that would violate and corrupt his daughter. In a covert manner, her dad allowed his daughter to be abused. If he had understood his role as a father to nurture, protect, and provide for his daughter, he would never have allowed pornography in his home. God, the Father, will protect and provide a safe environment for us if we yield to Him and allow Him to heal the wounds inflicted by an enemy that hates us. The Father will restore what the Enemy has stolen. He "satisfies the longing soul, and fills the hungry soul with goodness" (Psalm 107:9).

For the first time in her life, Julia felt that God loved her. She was able to connect her experiences as a child with her choices as an adult. Through repentance, understanding, and specific prayers to break the power pornography, promiscuity, murder, and self-hatred had over her, Julia was set free. As we all must do, she would daily appropriate what God had done for her through offering herself as a living sacrifice to the Father, choosing to trust Him, obey Him, and seek His way of living through His Word. We all must press on, as it says in Philippians 3, for the prize, by letting go of what is behind us and reaching out for what God has ahead for us.

TREAT THE ROOT PROBLEM, NOT THE SYMPTOMS

As she sat in my office on that first visit, we reviewed Julia's history, symptoms, and goals. In addition to being 100 pounds overweight, Julia also suffered with migraine headaches, irritability, severe PMS, heavy menstrual flow with cramping and nausea, anxiety, and insomnia. She had previously been diagnosed with fibrocystic breasts and suffered from frequent yeast infections. She had not taken the birth control pill for many years, but never felt "normal" since the abortion. Now she needed to get healthy and have a plan to lose the weight and strengthen what she had destroyed over the many years of self-inflicted dietary abuse. With such a substantial amount of weight to lose, we decided to break her plan into three-month segments and prioritize her goals. The first goal is always to ensure that the digestive system is working properly. I gave Julia a computerized symptom survey to complete. This survey helps to prioritize which systems need to be addressed and in what order. Julia's survey results revealed that her greatest need was digestive support followed closely by hormonal support for her pituitary gland.

It is important to stress that I don't treat a patient's symptoms. I take note of them and correlate them with the findings, but the care program is based on the results of the tests. So often people self-diagnose based on their symptoms. Even if they choose "natural" remedies from a health food store, they are still masking the true cause of the problem. Without a thorough evaluation, it is impossible to know what the root cause of a problem is, period. It's wonderful that the symptoms may resolve by taking a natural remedy, but in time the symptoms will return or create deeper imbalances that will show up in other systems in the body, making a true diagnosis more difficult. If this book awakens the knowledge that you may have similar imbalances, please check with a doctor who specializes in clinical nutrition before running off to the health food store to buy what may have worked for the people mentioned here.

An in-office zinc tally test revealed that Julia's zinc status was low. This is a very common finding. There are several reasons for zinc deficiency, but it is almost always seen with hormonal imbalances. Zinc is needed for the proper synthesis of progesterone as well as vitamins A and B_3. The zinc tally test determines

> The first goal is always to ensure that the digestive system is working properly.

zinc status in the body and is performed by having the patient hold about two teaspoons of the liquid zinc solution in the mouth for ten seconds. If there is no taste within that time period, the zinc status is low. If an awful bitter metallic taste is immediately experienced, the zinc status is sufficient. Zinc is needed for proper hydrochloric acid (HCl) production. Remember, HCl is the acid produced in the stomach to aid in the digestion of protein. Without it, food cannot be properly digested, causing stress to the pancreas and biliary system (liver/ gallbladder). For this we used Zypan and Multizyme.[2] Within three to four weeks her abdominal bloating was significantly reduced.

Next, we turned our focus to her pituitary gland. It was also determined that her thyroid and adrenals needed support, but since all clinical signs pointed to her pituitary, we supported it first. Quite often when the underdog gland is supported, the others balance more easily. To determine this, I performed a number of tests. One is called Ragland's test for postural hypotension. The blood pressure is taken with the patient seated, then again with the patient lying down. A third time, the cuff is inflated and the patient is asked to stand quickly. If the systolic pressure drops by ten or more mmHg, this indicates a need for adrenal support. Julia's initial blood pressure was 140/80. When she sat down, her blood pressure remained the same, but upon quickly standing it dropped to 120/80. This confirmed an adrenal issue.

Research by Elliot Abravanel, M.D., shows that there are body characteristics with each gland's malfunction.[3] While I do not support his work in its entirety,

I do see the body-typing characteristics to hold true in practice. With a weak pituitary, the weight distribution is around the stomach and upper back. He also noted that with this scenario, the person tends to crave salty, full-fat cheeses. Since her greatest area of indulgence was with cheeses and salty foods, this seemed consistent in Julia's case. When Julia first came to me, she looked bloated. She drank plenty of water, but always felt thirsty and seemed to be dehydrated. This was confirmed when I found her minerals, especially zinc, were quite depleted.

I was suspicious of her actual estradiol (estrogen) and progesterone levels. A woman's ovaries produce two hormones, estrogen and progesterone. Progesterone is needed in the proper amounts in order for estrogen to be produced. This process requires enzymes, vitamins, and minerals such as magnesium to do so properly. The ratio of these two hormones is very important, and subtle changes can trigger many symptoms. In a healthy menstrual cycle, estrogen levels rise in the first two weeks. Ovulation occurs, and then during the last two weeks of the cycle the ovaries produce progesterone. Just prior to menstruation, both hormones should decrease. If the pituitary is underpowered, progesterone production can be impaired. A female hormone saliva profile indicated that Julia's progesterone levels were exceedingly low. This could be the result of her diet or an imbalance set into motion from the birth control pills (which contain synthetic estrogens) years ago.

When progesterone is not adequate to oppose estrogen, a situation called estrogen dominance occurs. Estrogen dominance can occur due to a diet high in commercially grown fruits and vegetables, meats, and dairy products, due to the use of pesticides, hormones, and preservatives as well as from the exposure to petrochemicals. These are called xenoestrogens. Xenoestrogens compete for the same sites as natural estrogen. They have an estrogen-like effect on the body and are harmful because they act like estrogen in the body. These synthetic forms have been proven carcinogens. According to Dr. John Lee, "When estrogen becomes dominant and progesterone becomes deficient, then estrogen becomes toxic to the body."[4] Stress is the other non-dietary factor that can cause this. We are aware of the role the adrenals play in stress, but the pituitary gland has a definite role in trying to "put out the fires." Low progesterone may be the result of pituitary (LH) or thyroid insufficiency (which may be secondary to adrenal, anterior pituitary, or estrogen stress).

Natural progesterone is available over the counter in the form of wild yam cream. Though many advertisements say this can be used without a doctor's aid,

I highly advise against this. Even in this form, overuse or misuse can occur, so monitoring by a doctor is recommended. It is crucial to have someone with knowledge of how the hormones work to determine your need. I gave Julia a professional-grade cream containing herbs and nutrients that supports the production of progesterone. She would massage it on the skin of her stomach and breasts. I also supported her with a Standard Process product called Ovex. Ovex is not a hormone itself. It contains enzymes that help the body make progesterone as opposed to estrogen. Its phosphatase helps calcium assimilation and subsequently helps to prevent osteoporosis in two ways: hormonal support and improved calcium utilization. Ovex also provides vitamin E, which is important for steroid hormone production.

I wanted to see what impact supporting Julia's digestion and hormones would have on her weight. She dropped fifteen pounds in the first two weeks. Much of this was from fluid retention. Needless to say, we were excited, but this rapid weight loss would not continue.

> ## Healthy weight loss is no more than one to two pounds per week.

Healthy weight loss is no more than one to two pounds per week. Most of her symptoms subsided over the next month. Her eating plan was a tiered approach. Tier one was to eliminate the cheese and bad salt as well as all caffeine-containing items. She was to also avoid estrogen-producing herbs and foods such as fennel, anise, clover, milk thistle, sage, chamomile, dong quai, royal jelly, dates, apples, chickpeas, raspberries, carrots, and squash. Tier two was to add lots of green leafy vegetables and sea salt. (The brand I prefer is called Pacific sea salt.) She was allowed unlimited portions of vegetables, but no fruit for the first month. I didn't want to trigger any sugar cravings, so we kept these out until her blood sugar was stable.

She could eat an unlimited amount of any lean meat, fish, eggs, or poultry with her vegetables. Olive oil or butter used in moderation are the preferred fats for cooking. She would make salad dressing with organic apple cider vinegar or balsamic vinegar, flaxseed oil, and herbs of her choice. Literally hundreds of spices can be used once we open our creativity to these possibilities. Many people seem to think that salt and pepper are the only spices that exist. Indian spices such as curry, ginger, and cloves are wonderful and aromatic. Thai spices such as coriander, lemongrass, and chili peppers can be used to make chicken exotic beyond simply broiling it with salt and pepper. I encouraged Julia to buy some exotic food cookbooks that make vegetables and meats come alive. Some people don't know that there are a number of Italian recipes that don't include pasta. The wonderful spices of Italian cuisine include oregano, rosemary, and garlic. I love looking through exotic cookbooks and finding wonderful recipes that prove to the doubting mind that getting healthy can be fun and feel good.

Before my own family was convinced that eating organic, hormone-free foods could be delicious, I offered to cook the Thanksgiving meal for all the relatives. My mom asked me if I wanted it to be a potluck. I wondered why she would say this when I had for the first time in my life offered to cook an entire holiday meal. She was wondering who would eat my "kind" of food. She thought it would be bland and boring: steamed cabbage or something grotesque. I fooled them all. I pulled out all the stops and blew everyone away with a wonderful meal that was healthy and hormone- and chemical-free. My turkey was the best anyone had ever had. It's amazing how natural foods have so much flavor.

After the first month, Julia was allowed to have grapefruit with her breakfast omelet, but all the other restrictions remained. She was surprised at the energy she had and that she wasn't hungry. If she skipped a snack, though, she could feel it. By month six she was allowed to add one slice of sprouted whole-grain bread at her meal of choice.

SENSIBLE EXERCISE

What would a balanced program be without exercise? Exercise reduces estrogen production and improves circulation. I recommended Julia swim laps and cross-train by doing strength training and stretches with rubber exercise bands and an exercise ball. Thera-band is the most popular brand for both the bands and ball. Many books are available that teach how to do the exercises. Also, there are trainers at gyms who can instruct on the proper techniques. She also bought some Scripture memory cards to help her focus on God's Word. She would sit in a relaxed position, put on some soothing instrumental music, read, and meditate on the Scripture of the day. She did this for about fifteen to thirty minutes per day and used it as a time to lay her cares, concerns, and anxieties before the Lord. She had other times when she would worship the Lord and study the Word, but this time was simply to relax and meditate on God's Word as Joshua 1:8 admonishes: "This Book of the Law shall not depart from your mouth, but you shall meditate on it day and night, that you may observe to do according to all that is written in it. For then you will make your way prosperous, and then you will have good success." And good success she had indeed.

The first fifty pounds were her first big hurdle. She reached this and passed it in the ninth month. She would fall every now and then, but since she had worked through many of her emotional issues prior to starting the weight-loss program, there was nothing to pull the plug on her progress. Julia was happy for the first time in her life. It wasn't losing weight that made her happy, but knowing she was no longer a prisoner to her past and able to choose to lose weight because it was a healthier way of life for her. She wasn't doing it to please a man or to fit into any stereotype, but to be all God designed her to be. She wanted it all: the energy, vitality, real inner beauty, strength, and courage. She wanted the beauty Scripture speaks of: "But let it be the inward adorning and beauty of the hidden person of the heart, with the incorruptible and unfading charm of a gentle and peaceful spirit, which (is not anxious or wrought up, but) is very precious in the sight of God. For it was thus that the pious women of old who hoped in God were [accustomed] to beautify themselves" (1 Peter 3: 4–5 AMP).

Julia tore up those pictures from the days she served foreign gods, and chose to trust that as she remained committed to the truth of who she was, a beloved daughter of an awesome God, that He would continue to give her the strength to stay focused on His plan for her health, life, and future.

She is still taking off those unwanted pounds, and the person who has been buried beneath the weight has been revealed slowly but surely. As Rodin and Michelangelo could see the finished masterpiece before they chipped away even one

> She knows that whether she is 120 pounds or 220 pounds, she is beautiful.

speck of stone, our Father God sees, knows, and is faithful to complete the work He has begun in us. She knows that whether she is 120 pounds or 220 pounds, she is beautiful and no one can take that away from her. She chose to aim for a weight that would help her live a long, healthy life, physically able to do all she could to be Christlike in a world that isn't.

I know that Julia's life is similar to that of many women who have been prisoners of shame. Perhaps you were wounded as a girl by pornographic images that gave you the impression that your only purpose was to be a sex slave void of love and intimacy. Perhaps you didn't know until now why you have been unable to have intimacy with your husband or have been unable to sustain any long-term relationships. I want to encourage you. God is the originator of intimacy and knows what true beauty and romance is. Let's pray that the God who created the amazing colors of the rainbow and the sunset, the sweetness of a rose awakened by the morning dew, who opens the blind eyes and prison gates, can set you free from a hidden darkness of which you may or may not even be aware.

Awesome Father, many of your daughters have been violated and their virtue stolen by an enemy that would love to keep them from manifesting the beauty of your amazing love in their lives. We ask you, Father, to reveal yourself to each one of us in a way we have never experienced. Reveal the nurturing, protective, and providing aspects of your character to those of us who may have been raised by fathers not capable of raising us in the way you would have chosen. Father, help us to see what true beauty really is and how being loved with everlasting love feels. Give each of us strength to face the past and lay it at your feet. In Jesus' name. Amen.

And I am sure that God, who began the good work within you,
will continue his work until it is finally finished on that day
when Christ Jesus comes back again.

PHILIPPIANS 1:6 NLT

FIT TIP #14:

Exercise your spirit and mind. Buy or make Scripture memory cards and cuddle up in a cozy spot with some relaxing instrumental music to meditate on God's Word, asking the Holy Spirit to make it come alive for you.

FIT TIP #15:

Exercise your body with low-impact cardiovascular, fat-burning exercises. Swimming laps is an amazing workout that really trims the fat. Set a goal for the amount of time you will swim and then focus on doing more and more laps in that time frame. Later on extend the time until you reach a comfortable yet challenging workout. Water aerobics are available for those who don't really care for lap swimming. Meditate on the Lord and pray as you swim.

6 FIT AT FIFTY

Life-Saving Lifestyle Changes

Lisa left the hospital consumed with a multitude of thoughts and wondering what had happened to the account she'd been working on prior to being hospitalized. She realized this was a slightly distorted way of thinking; she ought to be grateful to be alive. As the hospital attendant wheeled her to the car, she told herself, *Time for a reality check. I've got to change the way I've been living.* Her husband, Carl, gently whispered in her ear, "Be patient, Lisa. Let's just take this one day at a time." For the last thirty years or more she had been on one track: working hard, resting little, and eating poorly. Carl was as supportive as he could be, although Lisa had a hard time receiving his love and support. This was a constant battle for her—one that several of her near-fatal experiences would soon change.

A few days later Lisa sat in my office, a bit nervous and afraid of what I was going to tell her she'd have to give up. Funny how that's what people immediately think of when they consult a clinical nutritionist. At her first appointment, however, I wanted to know about the events that led to the day Lisa thought was her last.

For the most part, Lisa had not realized the negative effects of her poor lifestyle management. She ran into various challenges through the years, some more serious than others, but none of them motivated her to change. Five years earlier she had had a scare with a lump she found in her breast. She tried to ignore it, but found it very painful around the time of her period and made a visit to her general practitioner for a checkup. A mammogram revealed some calcifications, and the doctor determined that she had fibrocystic breasts. She gave me a call at that time to see what I would recommend. I suggested cutting out the coffee, chocolate, black teas, and most junk food, and making sure her bowels were moving every day. She made it pretty clear that she just wanted some relief, was grateful that it wasn't cancer, and would consider making the dreaded lifestyle changes later when she had time. How many people wait to "have time"? We must make time, or our bodies will demand time, as Lisa found out the hard way.

A commercial lease broker, Lisa had been working on closing one of the biggest deals of her life. She was working what seemed like twenty-hour days for weeks and picking up fast food on the run, if she ate at all. Whatever was left in the office lunchroom—coffee, tea, donuts, or someone's leftover lunch from the day before—often was all she'd eat. This particular day she was the only one left at the office, combing through the final draft of the lease documents. Tired, she tried to push through so she could get home at a decent hour. She called Carl to let him know what time she'd be home, put the phone down, and got up to go to the rest room. As she stood, she felt lightheaded and faint. She staggered and had to lean against the wall. Instead of sloughing it off as no big deal as she had done in the past, she called 9-1-1. This time it was worse, and she was scared. When the paramedics arrived, she was sweating, short of breath, her pulse was erratic, and she felt pain in her chest. Lisa had suffered a heart attack. Unfortunately, she had a considerable amount of blockage and needed bypass surgery.

She joked and made light of all the events, but in her eyes I could see that this was the event that would define Lisa's life and destiny. Now fifty years old, Lisa tipped the scales at 202 pounds. For a woman 5'4" tall, this was just a bit out of the healthy range. As long as she and Carl had been married, his biggest complaint was that Lisa didn't cook. She preferred to eat out or order in. Her weight reflected this lack of dietary discipline, but she didn't care.

Lisa told me she had played tennis and run track in college. But after a while her work schedule consumed any time for sports. Carl made a good living and would have preferred that Lisa stay home so they could raise a family. But those dreams died early, as Lisa had it firmly embedded in her mind that she would never be a good parent. Besides, Lisa was afraid to trust her financial security in Carl's hands, let alone God's. Carl was an agreeable sort of man. He wanted to support his wife in her endeavors even though he didn't feel he had her equal support. He was not competitive, and eventually he let Lisa have her way and tried not to rock the boat.

Lisa shared with me some of her childhood memories. Her mother, much like herself, was not very affectionate and rarely expressed her love in any way. Her dad, a quiet man, similar to Carl, would gather the kids together late at night to raid the fridge or prepare some yummy dessert. She felt so loved in those moments. This to her was love. Her mom and dad fought constantly, or at least it seemed that way. Lisa and the rest of the family walked around on eggshells for fear that at any given moment Mom might be in a bad mood and blow a fuse. Her dad finally stopped talking to her mom or anyone in the house; he died quietly in his sleep at age sixty-three. Both parents battled with rage; one stuffed it, while the other, like an unpredictable tornado, destroyed anything or anyone in her path. Yet in her heart, Lisa still equated love with those moments with her dad late in the evening around the kitchen table. Unfortunately, Lisa also learned from her parents a very unhealthy way to deal with conflict. This bittersweet combination of passions fueled Lisa's drive and determination, bringing her great prestige and success but no joy.

Lisa knew what the Bible said about honoring her mother and father, but hard as it was to admit, she hated her mom, and she resented her dad for never standing up to her mother. Lisa made judgments and vows from that painful yet crucial time in her youth that not only affected her choice in a spouse but also established the foundation of what she believed love really was. Now she suffered because she could not support her husband and the goals he honestly felt God had placed within his heart. She tried with all her might to "Honor [her] father and [her] mother, as the Lord [her] God [had] commanded [her], that [her] days may be long, and that it may be well with [her] in the land which the Lord [her] God [was] giving [her]" (Deuteronomy 5:16). Because of the vows she had made as a child, she was still attached to her father in an unhealthy way, which in a sense was perpetuating her mom's behavior in her own household by not allowing her and Carl to be as one. Lisa couldn't submit to her husband and certainly could not receive his desire to support and take care of her.

This is such an amazing dynamic: the thing we least want we get. As we grow up, choices we made as children determine our choice of work, spouse, ministry, or extra-familial activities. The vows we make as children stick with us until we are brought to the cross of Calvary and are made aware of all that separates us from a full, intimate relationship with the Father through His Son, Jesus Christ. This is what eternity is, after all. Truly knowing the Father, the reason He sent His Son to die for us, and what our purpose is here on earth: to know Him, to receive His love, and to give it away.

John 17:3 tells us, "And this is eternal life: [it means] to know (to perceive, recognize, become acquainted with and understand) You, the only true and real God, and [likewise] to know Him, Jesus [as the] Christ, the Anointed One, the Messiah, Whom You have sent" (AMP).

Both Lisa and Carl came to have a relationship with the Lord while in college. Shortly after they were married, Carl knew in his heart that he was second to Lisa's dad. Lisa never learned how to love her husband, because she never saw love demonstrated at home in a healthy manner. She was never shown or taught what a man's role as a husband was to be or what a woman's role as a wife was to be. It was only her memories of Dad around the kitchen table eating desserts at night that told her she was loved.

We came to see it was this undercurrent that generated her cravings for snacks and sweets at night. She'd raid the refrigerator and gorge herself with whatever junk she could find. Lisa went to bed feeling loved and satiated, while her poor arteries were being clogged. Underneath was a resentment for her dad, weak men in general, and the domineering women they were married to; and ultimately she was buried in what she thought was her frustration with her weight and her life. I see this in my practice more than I would like to. A spouse will complain about the lack of support he or she receives from a spouse, but underneath there is some unresolved issue with a parent or a vow made never to be like that parent. This becomes the core of the health challenge, and until it is at least acknowledged, the health issue remains the same.

On one level, Lisa needed to deal with her childhood issues; but on a present level, she needed to change her diet and do whatever she could to prevent another heart attack. Lisa had had both a physical and an emotional heart attack. She was just plain worn out after fighting the battle on her own. She had never allowed her heavenly Father to take away the striving and struggling, because what would be left was her anger, self-hatred, and resentment for her dad and his own weakness as the leader of his household. These emotions kept a tight seal around her desire and ability to address the core issues of her health problems, and they were far too painful and too frightening to look at through human eyes alone.

> So few of us take God's Word in full faith, and we don't get those little hints He sends us.

The Lord brought Lisa, by allowing a crisis experience, to see that she really wasn't the captain of her own ship. So few of us take God's Word in full faith, and we don't get those little hints He sends us. Instead, we are driven to the cliff's edge of our experience, to the end of our self-dependency, where we can finally see God. While Lisa was in the hospital, the Father God began to do spiritually what the surgeons had done physically: give Lisa a new heart.

Wasn't this similar to what happened with the prophet Jonah? He had so much hatred in his heart; he actually wanted God to destroy Nineveh. But God takes the Ninevehs of our lives and turns them into a shepherd's field. He turns the place where we have hatred, the place where we were wounded, the place where we were not accepted, and turns it into a place of healing. Lisa had no idea how much bitterness, resentment, and anger she had pent up in her heart. She was working herself to death physically and emotionally. Like Jonah, Lisa wanted to die.

A HEALTHY HEART

The Master Surgeon had a tremendous amount of work to do in Lisa's heart, and I was commissioned to get it physically healthy again. Our to-do list included lowering her blood pressure and cholesterol, changing her diet, helping her lose fifty pounds, and getting her on an exercise program and a stress management program, while educating her on what it means to be truly healthy. We had a huge task in front of us, because this beautiful woman, as highly motivated as she was, was also very afraid.

Lisa's cardiologist had recommended she eat a low-fat, low-cholesterol diet and eliminate all salt, and that she take an aspirin per day and an array of medications, including a cholesterol-lowering drug. I would never tell a patient not to take a prescription drug. All I can do is share with her my opinion and allow her to decide for herself or allow her doctor to tell her it is no longer needed. My opinion regarding aspirin is rooted in research. Aspirin is recommended to help keep the platelets from clotting. But it also causes damage to the red blood cells that some researchers say is irreversible. The original research did show that aspirin helped to reduce the chance of having a second heart attack, but it was not found to actually prevent the incidence of having a first. Since Lisa had just had a heart attack, I wanted her to understand the big picture and offer tools to help her naturally prevent a second heart attack. Then she would be equipped to make decisions about her overall health rather than just using a drug that does not nourish the body and actually creates more deficiencies.

Dr. John Folts, of the University of Wisconsin School of Medicine, is one of the nation's leading researchers in cardiology. He is currently studying the anti-platelet/antioxidant properties of red wine, dark beer, fruit juices, and tea. He says, "These compounds appear to be better platelet inhibitors than aspirin."[1] And, less damaging, I might add. These items contain what are called *flavonoids*. Although Dr. Folts is studying these particular items, there are a number of healthier foods rich in flavonoids that are equally beneficial. Many people can't handle the caffeine in tea, and the sugar in alcohol is not beneficial either. It's not quite as pleasant to eat the white part of the orange peel, but this is a very high source of flavonoids.

Flavonoids naturally occur in most fruits and vegetables, especially in the buckwheat plant. It is unknown whether decaffeinated black teas offer the same benefit. Green and white teas have also been shown to offer incredible benefits. I don't know about you, but I don't have any buckwheat plants growing on my patio, and I can only drink so much tea. This being the case, most people find other ways to get the flavonoids needed to strengthen the heart. For example, I use two products to support every cardiac strengthening program: Cardio-Plus and SP Green-Food (both from Standard Process Labs). Cardio-Plus contains nutrients that support the strengthening of the heart muscle, and SP Green-Food is rich in rutin and bioflavonoids, made from organic buckwheat juice and barley grass juice. Because these products contain the synergists found in nature, they are more powerful than any synthetic fractionated product.

I also gave Lisa a magnesium supplement: Magnesium Lactate, from Standard Process. It has a relaxing and calming effect for high-anxiety personalities. Recent research in 22 patients (19 men and 3 women) who were between 43 and 69 years of age, showed that magnesium was found to reduce the severity of chest pain during a coronary spasm. There was a favorable response to the magnesium in 71 percent of those tested. The authors suggest that long-term oral magnesium supplementation may prevent or reduce coronary spasm in patients with angina pain.[2]

Lisa started on these whole-food supplements and added three to four table-spoons of omega-flo[3] flaxseed oil twice a day in a couple of ounces of pineapple juice. This makes it a bit more palatable for people who can't tolerate the taste. I also suggested she add it to some cottage cheese and use it on salads along with some organic apple cider vinegar. Flaxseed oil was a crucial asset in her healing process. This is an omega–3 fatty acid different from the omega–6 types found in cold-water fish. It has tremendous benefits for the heart, liver, skin, and brain. Sticky platelets indicate an omega–3 deficiency. Eskimos in Alaska have a surprisingly low incidence of heart disease even though their diets are very high in fat.[4] This tells me that fat is not the problem, but bad fats are!

I have noticed that in general people of blood types O and B can digest protein much easier and have little tolerance to grains and dairy products. Lisa's blood type was B, which in conjunction with her history led me to understand even more why her previous diet had caused her such distress.[5] However, anyone who lives on a fast- and junk-food diet will suffer from any number of symptoms or diseases.

> # It is impossible to put poor fuel into the body and not pay the price.

It is impossible to put poor fuel into the body and not pay the price. For some people this is realized in small ways, such as a lack of energy, while for others it shows up in the form of major degenerative diseases. It seems that one of the differences is the emotional factor. People who keep short accounts and effectively deal with the stressors of life seem to be less affected by the foods they consume. This is not to condone a poor diet for anyone, but it is amazing to see how a happy-go-lucky attitude contributes to longevity and vitality.

Lisa's diet was to be rich in green leafy vegetables, lean, hormone-free meats like lamb, fish such as salmon, eggs, butter, olive oil, flaxseed oil, and brown rice. I limited her fruit intake to a small serving of pineapple, apples, or papaya in the morning only. For breakfast she could have two eggs cooked in butter or a little olive oil with mushrooms and spinach or just soft-boiled eggs with a slice of toasted spelt (an alternative to wheat) bread or Essene bread. These breads are found at health food stores. She was to avoid caffeine and sugars at all costs. For her morning and afternoon snacks she could have raw vegetables with a small amount of real mayonnaise or unsalted nuts. Lunch included about three ounces of broiled fish over a large green salad with tomato, cucumber, red or green peppers, broccoli, celery, and other vegetables of her choice. For dinner, the same amount of protein (meat or fish), a cup of rice, preferably brown or wild, steamed or sautéed vegetables, one whole oat roll or one serving of Wasa-bread, and herbal tea. She could vary the types of meats and vegetables, and the portions of vegetables were unlimited.

If I were to use one word to describe Lisa's diet, it would be *balance*. It was my professional opinion that Lisa's core problem was not her heart but her lack of balance in every area of life. Her life was out of order. She needed balance at home, balance at work, and balance in her diet. Lisa had dieted twice in her life, once with her breast tenderness scare and then as a bet with some of the other people at work to see who could lose the

> People who keep short accounts and effectively deal with the stressors of life seem to be less affected by the foods they consume.

most weight by the holidays. She took a diet pill that contained ephedra (ma huang) along with eating vegetable broth subsidized by raw carrots, celery, diet soda, and lots of coffee. She felt as if her chest were going to explode. I'm surprised she didn't suffer a heart attack from the diet alone. She lost several pounds, but within two months after she returned to her "normal" way of life, she gained it all back and then some. The dietary balance Lisa needed included eating some of each food group in moderate portions at every meal.

Instead of placing her on a low-cholesterol diet, I placed her on a cholesterol-lowering diet. This may seem like a play on words, but they are two completely different concepts. A low-cholesterol diet is low in foods that contain cholesterol, namely eggs, red meats, and so on. But research is not consistent with this form of therapy. Rather, it is very consistent with eating whole foods that aid the body in naturally lowering cholesterol. Amazingly, it includes the same foods many cardiologists tell patients to avoid. Moderation is the key as well as the quality of the foods.[6] A cholesterol-lowering diet is consistent with research showing a null relationship between cholesterol intake and cardiovascular disease, morbidity, and mortality but a positive correlation with a balanced diet that promotes the balance of grains, fruits, vegetables, and animal products.

Contrary to commonly held beliefs, Lisa needed to add salt back into her diet. I can't tell you how many people believe that salt is bad. Most doctors and many nutritionists continue to tell patients that salt is bad—especially patients with high blood pressure. It is the common table salt that should be avoided, because it is simply sodium chloride. Many brands even add sugar and aluminum. This form of salt aggravates high blood pressure, because it interferes with the body's water balance. Many people who suffer with hypertension also suffer with edema (swelling). Sea salt is a whole product that contains all of the minerals and elements needed for healthy fluid balance.

In addition to using sea salt, it was imperative for Lisa to drink plenty of purified spring water. She was terribly dehydrated, so this combination proved quite helpful. Her urine was very concentrated and had a strong odor. With the addition of water and Celtic sea salt, Lisa's urine changed within days. Lisa never used to drink water. If she drank anything it was usually coffee or a soda. She jokingly said, "I drink plenty of water, it's just colored and bubbly."

NEW HEALTHY HABITS

Lisa actually embraced her new diet and began seeking counsel from her pastor to address her emotional wounds, anger, resentments, and self-hatred. I enjoy praying with patients and even helping them work through many of their emotional and spiritual issues, but I felt it was wiser for Lisa to take counsel from the pastoral counselors and prayer team at her church. Her pastoral counselor was also able to walk her through the various levels of healing needed in her marriage.

Lisa's home life was difficult for a while. Even though she was easier to live with since she had come home from the hospital, learning these new healthy habits was a new experience. She and Carl began to take slow walks together and even joined the local gym. The hospital had a facility that helped Lisa get started on her cardiac rehabilitation. Little by little her endurance and strength returned. Her rehab was slow, but she was committed. She and Carl signed up for a stretching class that had a strong emphasis on deep-breathing exercises. Similar to yoga, but without the non-Christian spiritual emphasis, this class was designed to improve circulation and oxygen to the brain and every cell in the body.

These exercises combined with her walks gave her the physical balance she had never experienced before. Along with eating five times per day, for the first time in her life Lisa experienced how "healthy" felt. One breathing exercise that I gave her is very simple and is done sitting in a chair. Sit straight with your shoulders square yet relaxed with your back against the chair. Place your hand on your stomach as you inhale slowly through your nose counting to ten and hold for a count of five. While you are holding the breath, focus on your abdomen to make sure it is extended as far as you can comfortably extend it. Exhale slowly. Try starting with five of these and work your way up to more, as you are able.

To help Lisa become aware of how she responded to the stressors of her life, we discussed how the body changes physiologically when under long-term stress. When someone experiences an event that is upsetting or surprising, the heartbeat and blood pressure increase, the palms may become sweaty, and breathing becomes more rapid. Concomitantly, emotions may be expressed with these physiological changes. Our bodies are designed to return to a state of balance within moments after the event has ceased. Health problems occur when the physiological changes remain long after the stressful event has subsided. We may not even be aware of how past events cause us to worry. But if the present situation does not warrant an increase in blood pressure, for example, chances are something from the past has yet to be resolved and the body is still holding on to that "memory."

Imagine someone holding a gun, preparing to take aim, and then pulling the trigger and shooting. After years of poor stress management, unhealthy diet, and lack of proper exercise, the body can constantly remain in this pull-the-trigger mode. It then takes very little to startle or anger that person. But just as the body adapts negatively to a constant state of stress, it can learn to respond to relaxation and change the physiology back to normal. With practice, you can reset your body's stress system. This is similar to reformatting a disk for your computer. Changes can be experienced both physiologically and emotionally.

> As the body is in distress it will give off warning signals that often go ignored.

In addition to the breathing exercise, I gave Lisa an exercise I call "body check." Periodically, she would pause and do a body check in which she would take note of her posture, level of comfort or discomfort, any aches and pains, tension in her shoulders or back, or any sensation of anxiety or uneasiness. So often in talking with patients, I find that people are completely disconnected from their bodies. They don't pay attention to how they feel. This is troublesome, because as the body is in distress it will give off warning signals that often go ignored. Many people are not in tune with the language of their body.

For example, after eating a meal, do you feel bloated? Do you ever feel lightheaded when you stand up quickly? Are you tired in the afternoons? These are a few of the warning signs the body may give us to say, "Hey, pay attention to me; I have needs that you are ignoring." Eventually its ignored whispers become shouts that will be acknowledged one way or another. But if we start to do "body checks" even a few times per week, we will notice how stress affects our body and our emotions at a point where we can do something proactive about it. Paying attention to your body periodically can reveal changes before they become problems. When you notice tension or discomfort, acknowledge it and do something about it. Maybe you just need to get up from your desk, walk outside, take a few deep breaths, or perhaps drink a cup of hot herbal tea to relax. But do something good for your body.

The other component in this relaxation process is becoming aware of mental stress. For Lisa, so much of her drive was motivated by anger. She never really stopped to think about how she felt or on what her attention was focused. She worried excessively and noticed a constant conversation going on in her head of things undone, done wrong, or forgotten. It wasn't until we started talking about relaxation that she even brought up the subject. She didn't want me to think she was crazy, but wondered if the constant "chatter" could be stress-related. She noticed it especially when working with new clients. She would have extensive conversations in her head, rehearsing her "lines" and preparing for any objections that might occur. The problem was that it did not stop at the end of the day. Late into the night, as she tried to sleep, the "chatter" would continue. I've seen a pattern with other friends and patients. Much of this mental stress seems to revolve around expectations in which there are five components:

1. *What did you want to happen?* This is what you expected. What you hoped in your mind or heart would happen. For example, Lisa hoped her potential client would like the large commercial space and make an offer.
2. *What happened?* These are the facts. Lisa's client wanted some time to think about it and told her he would call her in a week.
3. *Ideally, what could happen?* The client may or may not make an offer.

4. *How did you feel about what happened?* She felt discouraged and allowed the "chatter" of all the things she did wrong to play like an auto-repeat tape in her head.
5. *What did you do about it?* She then vowed to not allow herself to get too excited about new clients and instead be more reserved, while inside she was still afraid of being rejected.

Expectations are a huge force in our mental stress. Outside of God, we will process false expectations in one of two ways: either we will stuff them, or we will show them in a number of unhealthy ways. Ideally, we should surrender them, pray, or get prayer for these matters. We decided that Lisa would use her morning prayer and meditation time to deal with the potential "chatter" and surrender it to the One who holds our hopes. Psalm 42:5 comforts us, saying, "Why are you cast down, O my inner self? And why should you moan over me and be disquieted within me? Hope you in God and wait expectantly for Him, for I shall yet praise Him, my Help and my God" (AMP). Our hope and expectation are to be in God, and in Him alone are we to trust. When we have this quality of intimacy with Him, we can address that ceaseless "chatter" and tell it who is in charge of this temple.

Lisa made her to-do list each morning and wrote down all the issues left undone, and then she presented them to the Lord. She offered Jesus her to-do list every day and asked that He would not only lead her but that He would be Lord over her work and all the tasks and meetings of the day. This proved to be the most valuable meeting she would have each day. It quieted her mind, and by nighttime she was able to sleep with less "chatter."

Life looks amazingly different when we are no longer angry. As Lisa began to love and see herself through the Father's eyes, she discovered she saw everything differently. In 1 John 2:11, God's Word shows how living in hatred affects our perspective on everything. "But he who hates (detests, despises) his brother [in Christ] is in darkness and walking (living) in the dark; he is straying and does not perceive or know where he is going, because the darkness has blinded his eyes" (AMP). For Lisa, the heart attack and the revelations she experienced regarding her self-hatred were sufficient motivation for her to change her ways. We have more than sufficient evidence to let us know that our loving Father in heaven wants us to let go of anger, bitterness, and hatred if we want to live a full, blessed life.

Lisa's life experience spoke to me in many ways. I've heard it said that everyone has a hole in his or her heart, and only God can fill it. Lisa may have suffered a heart attack, but this was only the physical symptom of what had taken place in her soul many years before.

What about you? Has your heart been hurting, broken, or attacked? Have these wounds affected your relationships, your physical well-being, or your work? Have you or someone you love been through a "Lisa" experience? I know an amazing physician who specializes in open-heart surgery. He once told the prophet Ezekiel regarding the Israelites, in Ezekiel 11:19–20, "I will give them one heart—a new heart—and I will put a new spirit within them; and I will take the stony [unnaturally hardened] heart out of their flesh, and will give them a heart of flesh [sensitive and responsive to the touch of their God]. That they may walk in My statutes, and keep My ordinances, and do them. And they shall be My people, and I will be their God" (AMP). This is not only for the Jew but also for all those who are called by the name of Christ. Galatians 3:26 says that in Christ we are all sons of God through faith, and verse 29 reaffirms that if we belong to Christ, we are heirs according to the promise. Now, that's what I call great health insurance! We serve such an awesome God. He doesn't merely give us a Band-Aid to cover our wounds; He heals us from the inside out. If this is what you've been seeking, pray with me.

Awesome Father of all creation, I offer you my life as a living sacrifice. Forgive me for not honoring my parents. Forgive me for hating myself, the beautiful creation that you made with purpose and destiny from the foundation of the earth. Take my past, my wounds and my failures and my fears, and create in me a new heart. Give me eyes to see and ears to hear the still, small voice of your Spirit. Tear down the walls of division between those I love but don't always like and me, and help me to love them with your love. Thank you, Father, for healing me from the inside out. In Christ Jesus' name. Amen.

I will praise You, O Lord, with my whole heart; I will tell
of all Your marvelous works.

PSALM 9:1

FIT TIP #16:

Take a deep-breathing exercise class or look up information on how to breathe properly. Many excellent resources are available. In deep-breathing exercises, the focus is on effortless breathing. Don't force it; simply allow your body to relax. Perhaps you can imagine the Holy Spirit refreshing and renewing your body with His precious breath of life. Out with the old unhealthy habits and in with the new, which are only available by trusting the Father's path of life.

FIT TIP #17:

What did you learn about food from your parents? How was food used to celebrate in your home? Were you ever rewarded with food for good behavior? Were you ever sent away from the table for poor behavior? Journal what you learned about food from your childhood and note how these behaviors affect you now.

FIT TIP #18:

What did you learn about resolving conflict? How did your parents deal with their anger and frustrations? When you are angry, sad, frustrated, or hurt, do you eat, work, or shop? If none of these things, take some time to think about what you do when you experience these emotions, and journal your responses.

FIT TIP #19:

Take a moment out of each day and do a "body check" in which you pause and take note of how you feel, your posture, any tension in your neck or shoulders, any aches or pains, and do something about your observations. Whether that is standing and stretching, taking a walk, or having a cup of herbal tea, acknowledge your body and treat it lovingly, and it will continue to show you warning signs while they are still small and manageable. Perhaps your action step may be to call your doctor; but do something. Don't ignore the signals.

7 FIT FATALE

Battling Fear and Insecurity

"A perfect day" hung on the foyer wall at the television station where Erica worked. In a colorful antique tapestry, the sky was blue and every flower perfectly in bloom. Children ran to and fro over the countryside, and picnic baskets lay on blankets on the grass as ladies sat in their big-skirted dresses and sipped tea.

Erica was the envy of all her friends. She was young, exuding a free and loving spirit. In addition, she was very successful and her appearance always impeccable. I remember wondering, *Does she ever have a bad-hair day?* She had been on the fast track to success since high school, writing and memorizing goals since ninth grade. She knew what she wanted and what it was going to take to get there. Nothing and no one was going to stop her. What made her friends envious was not that she was successful, but that she was so nice. What was wrong with her? This package was too perfect. They knew what they saw on the surface, but what they couldn't see was the stress packed into this cute package.

Erica shared with me the industry "buzz" and the real deal behind the news, how anchoring wasn't what it used to be. She often told me how competitive the business had become, how the priorities were so conflicting, not to mention the pressure to remain young looking, thin, and attractive. There were so many people to please. Besides needing to look like a model, an anchor had to be flawless in the eyes of many people while maintaining originality. It was really tough. The anchor who looked good and who could touch the viewer with the most poignant story was the one who could gain the attention of her audience and keep it. Somehow Erica managed to live up to these lofty and incredibly unreasonable expectations and reveal a positive, beautiful, and confident tapestry. She was always trying to find the perfect balance.

At first, I wasn't privileged to know her dark secrets. When she initially came to see me, she pulled off a cool air. She gave me the typical plea about really wanting to be healthier, only later to reveal the "Oh, and, of course, I'd like to lose a few pounds" story. I hope I don't sound cynical, but after several years of practice I have seen so many people who are ashamed that their desire to lose weight is more important to them than being healthy. They tell me they want to get healthier, but once they lose those unwanted pounds, they drop out of sight. I wasn't sure if Erica would be that way, and I certainly was not about to assume so. I would let time and our appointments speak for themselves.

Every morning at five Erica was on the stair-step machine. Half an hour of fierce stepping was followed by half an hour on the treadmill. She watched the early news while sipping at least a liter of water. She said she felt good and just wanted to keep it that way. I don't remember what it was that broke the ice, but I do remember that she was almost embarrassed that I was able to see behind this beautiful tapestry.

When I was going through college, no one knew that I, an honor roll student, would binge on cookies and ice cream only to throw it up out of disgust. I didn't want a soul to know who or what I was really about. My façade needed to always look perfect, no matter how frazzled I was inside. Maybe my revealing this to Erica was what gave her the freedom to finally let her hair down. She knew I was a Christian, even though we didn't really talk about God at first. She made mention of a framed photo with a Scripture beneath it that I have in the office. The way she said, "I've read that one before" spoke to my heart; I wasn't sure about her relationship with God, but hoped to know more as I got to know her better.

Eventually Erica began to open up and tell me what was really going on inside. She shared with me the nights she would go home to a cold, empty house only to sit in front of the television with a half gallon of ice cream on her lap, watching her competition and comparing herself to the other female anchors. Did they look younger, thinner, smarter? Did they have a better sense of humor? Would they steal her viewing audience? Did they have a more stylish haircut? Was there a certain charisma about them? She tormented herself night and day with these and more questions. They were the standard against which she compared herself. I could relate to her frustration. When I was an intern in a clinic, it seemed the male interns were more respected than the female interns. It used to drive me crazy, and I would work harder to gain the respect of my professors as well as my patients.

Erica's frustration seemed to have begun about a year earlier when the pressure mounted just prior to a ratings sweep. The producer, in an honest attempt to motivate his crew, used other stations' anchors to compare to his group. He compared everything from their smiles and hairstyles to how they delivered their stories, even throwing in where they hung out in the mornings for coffee. He closed with "We need to be better, sharper, smarter, more articulate, and, of course, accurate."

What seemed like an innocent staff meeting was actually adding coal to the furnace of Erica's insecurities. Erica had grown up in a very active family. She had one older brother. They frequently went camping and enjoyed water sports, especially water-skiing. She led a pretty protected life, attending a private school and a local university. She did whatever she could to be her personal best, whether it was how long she could hold onto the water-skiing rope or winning a speech contest. She was committed to giving life her all. And she did. College kept her busy, so she didn't date much, but would hang out with the gang from her study group and enjoy a pizza every now and then. Leading a girls' Bible study at church was a great encouragement to her as well as to the girls. She loved teaching and being in charge as well as knowing she was serving the Lord. Maybe it wasn't the most noble of motives, but in the meantime she was happy.

Physically, Erica was tall and lean. When she was young, kids teased her, calling her a giraffe and other silly names. It didn't bother her too much at the time. Her confidence wasn't easily shattered back then. But she was never in the spotlight or compared to others as she was now.

Erica told me that now if she put on a few pounds, she would just go for a run a few times a week, and the weight would fall off within the month. Overall she kept very active and longed for summer when she and her family could go to the river or to the bay and ski.

In her heart, she had committed her life to the Lord. She read her Bible often and prayed. She admitted that most of her prayers were asking the Lord to help her get a job or a promotion, or to win a contest. Basically they were "do and have" prayers rather than "be" prayers. A "be" prayer is one that says to the Lord, "I want to be what you have designed me to be. I want to be in alignment with your will. I want to be who I should be to serve you more effectively."

CONFIDENCE IN GOD'S TRUTH

Erica was filling her need for reassurance with ice cream and her own commentaries about her competition. Before addressing her ice-cream challenge, she needed to address her spiritual issues. God wanted her to base her confidence in Him above everything else. Not only was her behavior unhealthy, it was also counterproductive. Every opinion we have of ourselves that contradicts God's opinion of us is a lie. Even if these opinions are negative and demeaning, they are still prideful. If we base our confidence on these distorted beliefs, we are exalting our opinion above God's. This is pride.

In Daniel 4, we find the story of King Nebuchadnezzar. He had opinions of himself that were beyond God's truth. God allowed his life to be reduced to that of an animal until he knew that God reigned over heaven and earth, and until he could see life from a godly perspective. He needed to know that what he had

> Before addressing her ice-cream challenge, she needed to address her spiritual issues.

was not of his own doing. Whether the belief in ourselves is egomaniacal or wormlike, the belief is still a lie. These are simply different faces of the same problem: pride. Just as a light bulb cannot express itself outside the connection with a source of electricity, we cannot function spiritually outside of our connection with the Father. As Erica tormented herself, she realized that she was magnifying herself above magnifying God in her career and in her health. Her opinion of herself was more important than what God thought of her. Doubt, fear, and despair in the spirit are what pain is to the body. The doubt, fear, and despair that I could sense in Erica's voice were warning signals of something deeper. She really didn't rely on God.

Most of Erica's success in life had come from her strong, intense commitment to hard work. She didn't have to rely on others too much. With this recent job stress, it seemed God was allowing her to see an area that she could not control. For the first time in her life, she felt out of control. Since she never had to rely on God for anything, she never really got to know Him. Hard as it was for her to believe, it seemed He was allowing the tapestry to unravel. This was scary for her. She realized she didn't know God well because she was so consumed with fear. Fear was what she served. It was her idol. She was in fear of losing her image, her job, and her perfect body; little by little God allowed her false beliefs to unravel. Her acknowledging this was the beginning of her healing process. This was God's priority.

This was illuminating rather than devastating. She knew that she could lose her job, but the joy of coming to really know and depend on God was encouraging to her. She could be freed from her prison of fear. Don't be mistaken, this didn't and doesn't always happen suddenly. For most of us these things are progressive revelations. But to the degree we are willing to believe and confess our unbelief, God is waiting to reveal His glory to and within us. The God that she was teaching in the Bible studies was now becoming real to her. She was able to move away from her fear and doubt and pride and be set free to experience the fullness of resurrection life.

You may be thinking, *This sounds good on paper, but how is it done practically?* By applying the Word of God. God tells us in His Word what the truth is. Our perspective of God determines how we interpret these truths. The places that need to die are also the places where we are unable to properly interpret the truth. As we take to heart the Word of God, we can look those dead areas in the face and speak the truth to them. Jesus is watching us, and He will not leave us to do any of this in our own strength. Not only is He there, He has given us the beautiful gift of the Holy Spirit.

AN APPOINTMENT WITH GOD

I gave Erica an exercise to do at home. Unlike sit-ups, this is a really tough exercise. I instructed Erica to confront her false beliefs in a two-hour appointment with God. She was to turn off the phone, radio, television, and any other distraction, and grab a box of tissues, paper, and pen. I suggested she pray before she began that God would direct her and give her true insight into what she believed about herself. For the first fifteen minutes she was to stand in front of her bathroom mirror (clothing optional) and look at herself. Really look at herself.

During the next thirty minutes she was to write down in detail every lie she thought about herself and spoke to herself. When we see these false beliefs on paper, it can be almost humorous, because some of them are so absurd. Yet we speak these lies to ourselves on a moment-by-moment basis. The next fifteen minutes of this releasing phase was to be spent in true repentance, asking God to forgive her for believing lies about herself. She was to say each one aloud, asking God specifically to forgive her for it. This is not to shame us but to put in proper perspective our position in our relationship with the Father. Here the seed falls into the ground and dies. When we die to our false beliefs, we allow the Spirit of God to awaken within us the truth of our identity. It was also at this juncture that Nebuchadnezzar's understanding returned to him.

The last phase is what I call the refueling phase. For the second hour, Erica was to comb the Scriptures and find God's truths to refute each false belief. Writing each of these out in full in the first person—using "I" or her name—would give her an entirely new perspective on God's Word. I encouraged her to write out what she sensed God was speaking to her heart. I said, "You may simply sense in the quietness of your spirit that He is saying, 'I love you.' Whatever it is, write it down and meditate on it until you fully believe it." It is extremely beneficial to summarize the truths that God speaks and write or print them out individually on paper and post them in plain view to be read at least twice every day. This reinforces the truth and provides ample fuel for the Enemy to be put to shame. An even more powerful method to cement the truth into our minds is to put these same statements on index cards and read them aloud several times per day. Talk about a powerful way to change the way we think. Unlike some repetitious mantra or positive affirmation, these are actual truths that God has written on our hearts individually.

It is important to know that once we are refueled, there are some dark forces out there that will want to immediately steal the good that has been planted in the soil of our souls. So we must be on guard and have God's truths handy so we can fling some truly powerful darts back when we feel vulnerable or feel that we are being attacked.

After this life-changing experience, Erica found she had a new perspective not only of herself but also of God, her work, and her nighttime binges. They stopped. The void was no longer calling out to be filled by something empty. She was now filled with that which truly satisfied—the love and intimacy of the Father. I gave her some basic health-enhancing nutritional advice that she was easily able to implement into her life. The main nutritional recommendation was to not purchase any unhealthy snack foods, especially ice cream. If her environment was safe, she was more likely to calm herself and review her biblical truths than to give in to the momentary temptations. Every time she went to the grocery store, she was to stock up on healthy alternatives. Since she had been eating ice cream, I suggested she freeze berries or grapes to have as a healthy snack when she wanted something sweet. This was an easy transition, and, best of all, it made her happy.

Even though Erica had been gaining weight, the fuel for her true and permanent weight loss rested in the reversal of her false belief system. The tapestry remained beautiful on the outside, but God did some major repairs on the reverse side. Sometimes we judge others or ourselves by what we see. The picture looks pretty, and we assume that person has a problem-free life. Know that God is working on all of us, and though we don't want to assume that everyone has deep issues, we also should not assume that just because the tapestry looks perfect, that beautiful person is not struggling.

Maybe Erica reminds you of yourself or of someone you know. So much energy and effort are put into finding the right diet, when the answer is there all the time in the person of Jesus Christ. Hard as it may be to believe, He does care about the small things as well as the big things. If it concerns you, it concerns Him. Let's pray:

Father of all truth, infinite wisdom, and knowledge of every detail of my being, I confess that I have believed the lie. I have believed things about myself that contradict your Word. I want to know the truth and be set free. Today I lay my life down and ask you to show me the false beliefs about you, about others, and about myself that are keeping me from living the resurrection life you have prepared for me. I thank you for loving me and teaching me to love myself and to love others. In Jesus' name I ask these things. Amen.

Strengthen me according to Your word. Remove from me the way of lying, and grant me Your law graciously. I have chosen the way of truth; Your judgments I have laid before me.

PSALM 119:28–30

FIT TIP #20:

Take two hours and do the exercise described on page 94 and 95, which will help you see yourself as God sees you. The Lord will lead you to see the false beliefs, repent of them, and be filled with His truth.

FIT TIP #21:

Don't buy unhealthy snack foods. Keep your environment safe, healthy, and pure. For example, keep fresh or frozen berries or grapes on hand for a sweet snack. If it's in the house, you will eat it.

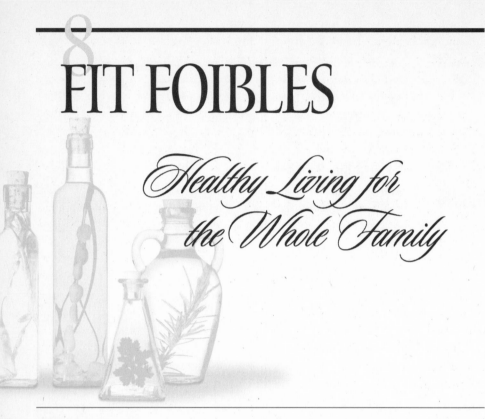

8 FIT FOIBLES

Healthy Living for the Whole Family

Karen sat in the emergency room with her two-year-old daughter, Laney, for the third time in a year. Over an hour had passed since she'd signed in, and their name was yet to be called to see the doctor. Karen was a wreck. Though she had a great job, she knew there was only so much her boss would tolerate. She had already used her vacation days as well as all of her sick time, due to one catastrophe or another at home. If Laney didn't have an ear or sinus infection, one of the other girls was sick with a cold or was suffering with one of their many allergies. There was "something" to deal with every week.

Karen wanted so much to keep the girls healthy and to feed herself and her kids well, but it seemed that whenever she made honest attempts at changing things, something would happen. Since her divorce, she'd gone from a size 8 to a size 14. She would cook meals at home if she had the time, but she was too tired to add to her list of Mommy-do's. She didn't sleep well and seemed to always be running on empty. The girls spent every other weekend with their dad. This was Karen's only time to catch up on errands and housework. Her ex-husband paid alimony and child support, but wasn't about to lose a day of work to take the girls to a doctor's appointment.

At our first appointment, she said it seemed as though she hardly ate anything but felt bloated all the time. In spite of her relatively low caloric intake, she continued to gain weight. She was so distracted by the stress of her life that her focus was more on the cares of this world than on seeing the "goodness of the Lord in the land of the living" (Psalm 27:13). This "treadmill" life, I believe, is an intentional diversionary tactic of the Enemy. If he could keep her focused on her children's poor health, her weight, job stress, and finances, he could keep her immobilized and deterred from the path that God had for her. As she saw how she was being assaulted, she felt sad and a bit distraught. At that moment it was hard for her to believe life could be any other way.

Isaiah 61:1 gives an encouraging word and a promise of freedom to those who are distraught and bound. "The Spirit of the Lord God is upon me, because the Lord has anointed and qualified me to preach the Gospel of good tidings to the meek, the poor and afflicted; He has sent me to bind up and heal the brokenhearted, to proclaim liberty to the [physical and spiritual] captives, and the opening of the prison and of the eyes to those who are bound" (AMP). Doesn't this verse fit the situation? So often we look for solutions on the same level as the problem instead of looking first to the spiritual realm to find God's solution. God's solution is always based on God's purpose. His plan is most easily implemented by our first being obedient to following what Matthew 6:33 says: "But seek for (aim at and strive after) first of all His kingdom, and His righteousness [His way of doing and being right], and then all these things taken together will be given you besides" (AMP). I add "most easily," because sometimes many of us have to learn God's purpose the hard way. I certainly have.

I think the Father smiles when His children willingly submit to Him and ask for wisdom. Karen's desires and intentions were good, but she was going about it all in her own strength. She wanted to eat right, cook healthy meals, and improve her kids' health, but she didn't know how to transition from her existing methods to healthier, more productive ones. Until now she didn't see her challenge as first a spiritual one. She loved God and fully desired to serve Him. Now God was beginning to show her what being a co-laborer with Him really meant. Just because someone is not living in blatant sin doesn't mean she is truly seeking God first. Karen thought she needed to "get her act together," while God was saying, "Give your act to me, and we'll get your act together."

I've encountered so many moms in this situation. It's such a Catch-22. Their time is so consumed with dealing with family health issues that they don't have time to be healthy. Many can relate to working so hard to hold "it" all together that they don't have time to live, feeling that they are climbing an endless ladder that's leaning against the wrong wall. There seems to be so much fear in entrusting their family's health and weight issues to God. But fear will not take us to the path where God is leading us.

> God was saying, "Give your act to me, and we'll get your act together."

Healthy living is like a forbidden zone that I sense many Christians are afraid to venture into. They may ask for prayer when they or loved ones are sick, but to actually think that many of their challenges could be prevented is a foreign concept. If up to 85 percent of our health challenges are caused by our lifestyle, then many of us have a wake-up call coming. The children in our society are suffering needlessly. Their ailments range from frequent infections to hyperactivity, and they are given one medication after another. Childhood obesity and diabetes are also on the rise. I know many Christian women taking anti-anxiety and anti-depressant medications. I want to let them know that perhaps some of their family's as well as their own symptoms and health problems could be lifestyle-related. There is no judgment placed on people who are taking medications. However, if they choose to ignore the path that could help prevent or correct the cause of their challenges, then it becomes a spiritual issue rather than a medical one.

I use homeopathic remedies in my practice. According to homeopathic philosophy, spiritual and/or emotional illness is the highest and deepest form of disease. I think it's ironic that an ancient healing art such as homeopathy agrees with God's Word. Even in Oriental medicine, much attention is given to addressing the emotional imbalances as a part of restoring health and vitality. I believe we can take some of these alternative principles and find scriptural validation for them. Simply put, when we are out of alignment spiritually, everything else will subsequently be out of alignment. I was recently given a copy of Pastor Henry Wright's book *A More Excellent Way*.[1] I was amazed at how this book so clearly showed the spiritual and emotional components to disease. This is exactly what I have been sharing with my patients for years.

STRATEGIES FOR CHANGE

The Enemy uses a variety of distractions or diversions to thwart God's plan for our lives. If he can keep us focused on our weight, having a mate or not, our low self-image, or our children's health, we can't focus on what's most important: the kingdom of God and His will for our lives. It's a simple strategy, and unfortunately it's working. It is very discouraging to have kids who are always sick, when Mom is too tired to effectively deal with it. But the Word of God encourages us when it says, "Casting the whole of your care—all your anxieties, all your worries, all your concerns, once and for all—on Him; for He cares for you affectionately, and cares about you watchfully" (1 Peter 5:7 AMP). Not only does God know, care, and see, He also wants to be an active participant in every detail of the solution. This is so encouraging in a confusing world. We don't have to do it alone.

For a single mom there is so much pressure. Karen was no different from many in her situation; though she knew Jesus, she often found herself frustrated as she trekked the "Mom path" alone. She sometimes felt like God's stepchild, moving forward even when she thought God didn't care. God did care for her, and He wanted to show her a multifaceted strategy.

Instead of focusing first on Karen's weight issues, we decided to turn the focus on health, sharing ways to help her family become healthier. This way her children would have fewer health problems, and she could rest and keep her job.

A balanced body will naturally reach an optimal weight.

As a bonus, she would lose weight in the process. I think my theme slogan has become "A balanced body will naturally reach an optimal weight." In Karen's case, her only real food issue was in not knowing what to buy or cook, along with being too busy or tired if she did know. This was a project that would take time and planning. With our goal in mind, we set out to accomplish this seemingly monumental task.

First, I needed to assure Karen that she did not have a weight problem. She had a knowledge problem. Her weight gain was merely the result of her not eating properly. There were no real hormonal or digestive imbalances—yet. If she were to continue in this lifestyle, though, she would develop these imbalances or more serious health problems. But thankfully they had not occurred yet. Her schedule was so hurried that she usually ate the fast foods that she fed her kids. These meals consisted of high, poor-quality fat and highly processed, nutrient-poor foods. What seemed like an impossibility was indeed possible, especially now that God was at the center of our endeavor. Her daughters already were heavier than other little girls their ages. We knew that if she continued in her current behavior, Karen's daughters would probably become obese, and eventually the problem would be more than one of knowledge.

Karen's first assignment was to keep a journal of her children's and her activities. For one week she was to write down everything they did from the time they woke up to the time they went to bed. She would need to employ the talents of her kids in accomplishing this task. Once she completed this first assignment, Karen saw that after the nine hours blocked out for commuting and work, she had about four hours per weekday to spend with her family and to accomplish household tasks.

The second assignment was to buy a dry-erase board and make a chart for each day of the week. Along the left border, Karen wrote all the "majors" that needed to be accomplished each week. Each had a colored marker assigned so they could clearly see which chores were theirs. The majors included Karen's job, her commute, sleeping, eating, cleaning, laundry, and helping the girls with their homework.

Taking all of this into consideration, Saturday became the most important day of the week for Karen. On Saturday mornings she would sit down and write out the schedule for the coming week, blocking out mandatory activities. Then she did something she had never done before: She planned her meals, grocery shopping, and cooking for the week. She wasn't a bad cook, but she had developed some bad habits. Every Saturday morning she would commit to this task and commit it to the Lord. Meal planning is a discipline that saves so much time it's unimaginable, until you try it. Good-bye to spur-of-the-moment stops at the convenient fast-food restaurant. Next, we factored in how the kids could help out. Kristen and Alexa were seven and eleven years old. Two-year-old Laney wasn't much help at first, but the older girls traded off caring for her, while Mom focused on the meal planning. Karen even spent one morning teaching Kristen and Alexa how to sort and do the laundry. It turned out to be a tremendous help.

With their shopping guidelines in hand, they all went to the local farmers' market (available year-round in Southern California) and to the health food store. They bought fresh produce from the farmers' market and their meats and dairy products from the health-food store. Once every two months they stocked up on toiletries from the bulk-shopping superstore. The girls loved these outings. It was a rich educational experience that they grew to look forward to versus spending Saturdays in front of the television. I explained our plan to them, and they saw how valuable their help was and gladly pitched in.

Once Karen got in the rhythm of managing her time more efficiently and rallying the support of her daughters, we focused on what foods to eat, what to eliminate, and how to make meals as healthy as possible. The rule of thumb is "fresh is best." The fresher the food the more nutrient-rich it will be. As Karen went through her kitchen cabinets, she realized that many of her staples were highly processed boxed, canned, or bagged items. There were three levels of this health transformation. Level one was to quit the absolutely bad habits, such as eating at fast-food restaurants. Level two involved learning to eat healthy, balanced meals rich in fruits, vegetables, and whole grains; and level three added fresh, organic homemade foods.

NEW HABITS, BETTER CHOICES

What is the difference between organic and commercial foods? Over the last fifty years or so there has been a tremendous decline in the nutrient density of commercially farmed produce. A group of organic farmers in California, having tested some of their produce, found it much higher in many vitamins, especially vitamin C. One study in particular at a U.S. Department of Agriculture research facility looked at the published comparisons of organic versus conventional crops.[2] The results showed that organic crops had, on average, up to 30 percent more vitamin C, iron, magnesium, and phosphorus and significantly less nitrates. There were trends showing higher levels of nutritionally significant minerals, lower levels of toxic heavy metals, and better protein composition in organic as compared to conventional crops. From nutritional value to environmental value, organic farming's benefits far outweigh its slightly higher costs. There are many other benefits as well. Some of them have a direct impact on human health—such as cleaner water and the absence of pesticide residues. Other benefits are more related to the environment as a whole.

Organic produce may be difficult to find in some areas, but it is becoming increasingly more available. In most cases only produce that is in season will be available organically. I recommend freezing produce (to maintain freshness) for use when it is out of season.

Back to Karen and her newly empowered team. They would buy their groceries for the week on Saturday, then spend time cooking together while listening to music, laughing, and sharing with one another on a new level of intimacy. Everyone participated—even Laney—whether in stirring soup, tearing lettuce, or peeling bananas. The foods were then either frozen or placed in containers in the refrigerator and labeled for the day they were to be used.

Karen and her daughters had a bit of adjusting to do, because their taste buds needed time to adapt to the more natural foods. This didn't take long, because Karen had managed to convince the girls that they would all feel better in the long run. By Saturday evenings they were pooped and would often nestle up together on the sofa to watch a movie. Whereas before Karen did all of the work, they now grew closer to one another as they learned to run a household as a family.

After they got the hang of this new way of living, the next level was to invest in some small kitchen appliances. When you are looking to make healthy meals, the optimal solution is to invest in healthy cooking appliances. The three I would recommend to purchase first are a grain mill, a high-powered blender, and a food processor. They don't all have to be purchased at once, of course, but a grain mill would be my first choice.

Using a grain mill is more important than having a bread machine.

Grains are very inexpensive. When you compare how much could be spent in a year on fast foods and store-bought breads, it is clearly less expensive to bake your own. Using a grain mill is more important than having a bread machine. A grain mill gives you fresh flour that has all of the nutrients still in it. Making fresh bread from processed flour isn't really that healthy. It's the freshness of the flour that is of greater importance. You wouldn't beat an egg, leave it on the counter for a week or two, and then cook it and serve it as a fresh egg. When grain is milled, the oils begin to spoil or go rancid. This is why bread companies enrich their products. Enriching basically removes the aspects of the grain that would spoil. Over thirty different vitamins are destroyed in this process and replaced with a few. If a whole grain is milled and utilized within forty-eight hours, all of the nutrients are left intact. Whole grains are a rich source of vitamin E and the B vitamins. Isn't is amazing how the nutritional specialists tell us to take these vitamins to protect our heart and reduce stress, when if we ate what God provided for us in the form of whole grains, we wouldn't need to take anything extra?

The *quality* of the foods we eat is more important than *what* we eat. This aspect of a healthy eating transition is probably the most important, in my opinion. Understand that eating whole foods is not the norm and will be considered by many to be unnecessary or even crazy. I assure you it is neither crazy nor abnormal. We have been duped as a society into thinking that all the fast and processed foods are no different from whole foods, and all the synthetic vitamins that fortify and enrich these foods are harmless. This is far from the truth. Some think that people who eat organic foods also burn incense, wear patchouli oil, and live in a commune. How many times have we referred to someone who eats whole, organic foods as a "health nut"?

In a world that seems upside down spiritually and physically, being healthy is often viewed as odd and eating junk and fast foods is considered normal. It was probably similar in Daniel's day. Daniel had made a commitment to God that he would not eat the fine foods of the king. But the chief of the eunuchs feared that he would lose his head if the king were offended by Daniel's appearance. He assumed that if Daniel and the three other young Israelites didn't eat the foods of the king, they would look sad and unhealthy. Daniel challenged the chief by requesting that for ten days he and his friends be allowed to eat only vegetables and legumes. He wanted the eunuch to compare the appearance of him and his friends with the other youths. Not only did they put on weight but they also looked better than the other young men.

The point I'm trying to make is not a scriptural sell on vegetarianism, but rather how a society can put pressure on us to conform when logic and thought don't back the reasons why we should conform. Our society accepts mediocrity in health and even goes so far as to call this substandard life normal. It seems to me that those foods that are healthy should be the minimum standard, and we should not have to go to a special store to purchase them. I find it humorous that we have what we call "health food stores." Does this mean that the other stores are "unhealthy food stores"?

My goal with Karen was to help her change some of the destructive behaviors that were consuming not only her time but also her family's health. Again, I stress, these changes do not occur overnight. It takes weeks and even months to break old habits, but with the power of God anything is possible. As Karen learned to focus her energy on God first, she found that her role as a mom became much more enjoyable. By eating better, she had more energy to be available for her girls. This was a rich and rewarding opportunity of growth for the whole family. Over a six-month period this household lost a tremendous amount of extra weight, and they had fewer doctor's visits for colds, infections, and allergies. This was a true blessing, since this is where much of Karen's time was lost, not to mention her job security.

Karen's situation is very likely similar to that of hundreds and even thousands of women. Rather than looking at how big your problems are, take a moment to ask your Father to show you how big He is. If you can get a glimpse of how big He is you may be able to have the faith to believe He can take care of your problems too. Pray with me that the Father may impart to you such vision:

> *Father, how great you are and how you love us in ways we cannot comprehend. I ask you in Jesus' name to give us bigger eyes to see you as you really are but also to see the diversions of the Enemy. We know that the more we focus on you the less we can be diverted by the devil. We long to let you out of the cramped box we keep you in and to change our limited opinions of you. Help us to believe that you not only love us but you are there with us as we raise our children. Help us to believe that you will enable us to do our part in improving their health. Give us strength, courage, and endurance to make the necessary changes for this transition to occur. We bless you and thank you. Amen.*

Be careful! Watch out for attacks from the Devil, your great enemy. He prowls around like a roaring lion, looking for some victim to devour. Take a firm stand against him, and be strong in your faith. Remember that Christians all over the world are going through the same kind of suffering you are. In his kindness God called you to his eternal glory by means of Jesus Christ. After you have suffered a little while, he will restore, support, and strengthen you, and he will place you on a firm foundation.

1 PETER 5:8–10 NLT

FIT TIP #22:

Take a trip to the grocery store and buy tasty, healthy foods. Based on what you can afford, start buying healthier ingredients to cook with. Maybe you can replace one unhealthy choice per week, maybe more. Whatever you are able to do, commit to it. For example, purchase sparkling water instead of soda, Stevia (a natural herbal sweetener) instead of your usual sugar substitute, or frozen or fresh berries or grapes in place of ice cream.

FIT TIP #23:

Include your children in your "get healthy" campaign. Making them active participants educates them as well as reduces the stress of your doing it all on your own.

FIT TIP #24:

Make a meal plan and shopping list before you go to the store. This way you are less tempted to buy impulsively.

FIT TIP #25:

Start shopping at local farmers' markets. Many of the farmers offer produce free of pesticides and genetic modification. The prices are usually reasonable, and since the markets are usually set up outside, it's a good opportunity to get fresh air as well as experience shopping the way our ancestors probably did.

9

IT DOESN'T FIT

When Self-image Is Based on a Lie

"No one wanted to hang out with the fat girl. Everyone in my school was thin, the primary obsession being which sorority to rush." These are the words Alicia used when she shared with me about the time she came to accept that being heavy was just her lot in life.

"I was always the funny one, the one people could talk to, the one they used as a watchdog when they were doing something they didn't want their parents to know about." Alicia had been overweight her entire life. During college she stopped dieting and conceded that this was the way it would always be. A doctor once told her it was hereditary; she would always be heavy. Now her health was becoming compromised, and her weight needed to be addressed. Her medical doctor told her that her blood pressure was too high, and she needed to make some diet changes, add exercise, and try to lose some weight. This is what brought her to me.

I sat and wondered who this wonderful woman truly was. What was going on inside her heart, her head, her body? Beyond wanting to give her a printout of dietary do's and don'ts, I needed to understand her beliefs about herself and support her from this perspective first. Matthew 19:19 tells us that we are to love our neighbor as ourselves. I wanted to understand how Alicia saw herself and just how different that was from what God says about her. When I notice an acceptance or complacency in a patient regarding an unhealthy situation, I can't help but wonder what contributed to this attitude. In this case, I wondered what might have occurred in her childhood to alter her self-image. Even if from her youth she was told that being big was her plight, there was something that could be done not only to improve her health but also to improve her fixed outlook on life. She never felt valued for who she was as an individual.

There is a fine line between accepting who you are and being complacent or unwilling to change. Self-acceptance brings with it a confidence that is God-given. There is peace in knowing you are just where God wants you to be, what He wants you to have, and what He wants you to do. Complacency is sin because it is an acceptance of less than God's design for you. It is self-perspective based on circumstances and the opinions of people. Without digging deeper into the core of her being, it could be easily missed that Alicia's self-acceptance was rooted in a lie.

After her visit to her physician, she knew she needed to lose weight no matter what she had been told in the past. She was 5'3" and weighed 190 pounds. She had a huge appetite and loved all the wrong foods. She cooked many meals as she had since childhood. She did most of the cooking then because her mom was often ill and her parents relied on her to take care of many of the household duties. Her brothers helped a bit, but for the most part she took care of the house. When she went off to college, she still cooked but had a difficult time adjusting to cooking for one person. She was also very lonely even in the midst of a huge university.

Alicia needed her mother, but her mom wasn't physically or emotionally available. Unfortunately, this left a young girl with adult responsibilities and no one to nurture her and provide the support, love, wisdom, and guidance that might help her mature into a healthy young woman. Her feelings of insignificance allowed the Enemy to have an anchor in her soul that kept her down. She had no one to comfort her when she felt insecure and alone.

As a very young girl, she had had no one to dry the tears when she wasn't invited to the school dance—no one to understand when the kids at school teased her and called her "Miss Piggy" or "dough girl." She was not aware that God was there, holding her, comforting her. She didn't recognize or acknowledge

Him. Alicia needed a release valve to ease the pressure of all the internalized stress from running her childhood home. She never got to actually *be* a child. Nor did she receive focused attention from her mother so as to be properly nourished emotionally. She used food as her release valve and believed being overweight was just the way she was made.

> ## She used food as her release valve and believed being overweight was just the way she was made.

As the lame man lay at the steps of the Beautiful Gate, he too accepted his plight as he stretched out his hand for help. Day in and day out he was laid on the steps of the temple, never thinking it possible to actually enter in. No one who was lame was even allowed in such a holy place. I imagine he wondered what it would be like to jump and dance, walk and worship as others did. Many days he probably fantasized about it but never believed it could be possible. Yet with innocence and expectation in his eyes, he sincerely asked for a handout. His daily provision would not be from God but from the passersby as they entered the temple. Many ignored him. Some pitied him. Others were bothered by having to step over him or around him. Yet this man at the Beautiful Gate persisted—until one day John and Peter walked by.

Certainly it was not the first time they had seen him, but it was the *right* time. The time appointed by the Holy Spirit to lay this man upon their hearts. He had probably been put there every day since he was a child. Begging was his nature, his character, the "way he was." Yet Peter and John turned his focus from having his temporary need met and momentary cup filled to being completely healed and refreshed by God Almighty. In Acts 3 we join in this miraculous transformation:

> One day Peter and John were going up to the temple at the time of prayer—at three in the afternoon. Now a man crippled from birth was being carried to the temple gate called Beautiful, where he was put every day to beg from those going into the temple courts. When he saw Peter and John about to enter, he asked them for money. Peter looked straight at him, as did John. Then Peter said, "Look at us!" So the man gave them his attention, expecting to get something from them. Then Peter said, "Silver or gold I do not have, but what I have I give you. In the name of Jesus Christ of Nazareth, walk." Taking him by the right hand, he helped

him up, and instantly the man's feet and ankles became strong. He jumped to his feet and began to walk. Then he went with them into the temple courts, walking and jumping, and praising God. When all the people saw him walking and praising God, they recognized him as the same man who used to sit begging at the temple gate called Beautiful, and they were filled with wonder and amazement at what had happened to him. (Acts 3:1–10 NIV)

What was true of this lame man was true in a sense of Alicia. She continually waited at the "temple gate." She was satisfied with "just enough," when "more than enough"—complete healing—awaited her. Day by day her cup was filled, simply by being included. She had a sense of humor, was helpful, and was not a threat to anyone. She found this satisfying, yet it was only a substitute for true happiness, fulfillment, and holiness. She began to resent those who filled her cup and desired those who did not. Instead of entering into the temple and experiencing true intimacy with the Lord, she hung out on the steps, trying to get her cup filled with the affirmations and acceptance of people. Day by day her soul eroded, while the cup the Lord wanted to fill remained empty. Desiring people to feel sorry for her or to accept her just enough to fill her cup and make her feel okay for the day are not the attitudes of one who lives in true fellowship with the Lord; they are the attitudes of a victim. Because when tomorrow came, Alicia would be back with her empty cup, needing to be filled again.

Some of us have a hard time trusting God to fill our cup. We medicate our emptiness with food, alcohol, sex, or other more addictive agents. But if we really knew Him, we would know that He does provide for every need. To put it another way, we can rest in the maternal nature of the Father as we allow Him to nurture and care for us. As a baby nestles against its mother's bosom, so the Father wants us to rest in the bosom of His care. This is true intimacy.

Alicia missed this resting stage in her childhood development. Not having sufficient parental nurturing, she self-medicated with food. She rationalized her appetite by saying she was made that way. Knowing why things happened in our past doesn't make them go away. We need to take the information and prayerfully consider how the Lord would have us act to bring about true healing.

OVERCOMING BITTERNESS AND RESENTMENT

The first area Alicia needed to address was the bitterness and resentment she held against her mother. Hebrews 12:15 says, "See to it that no one misses the grace of God and that no bitter root grows up to cause trouble and defile many" (NIV). Alicia needed to forgive her parents and ask the Lord to help her release them from her judgment and dishonor. She loved her parents, and at first didn't realize she held them in judgment. Though they had done the best they could and truly loved her, she did not receive the nurturing, guidance, and protection she should have had. When she forgave them, she could accept the forgiveness Jesus had already provided. This step allowed Alicia to move forward for the first time in years to address the food addictions she had developed. Most of us can admit to areas in our past that we need to face. The reality is that often we don't face them, and that is why so many suffer from addictions—whether mild or severe. There are very few people who don't have something they use to self-medicate.

The next area Alicia needed to address was to allow her heavenly Father to establish His throne in her heart. Now that all the bitterness was gone, there was room for the true God to move in. She asked the Father to make her heart His home and to establish the kingdom of God in her life. Romans 14:17–18 says, "The kingdom of God is not a matter of [getting the] food and drink [one likes], but instead, it is righteousness—that state which makes a person acceptable to God—and heart-peace and joy in the Holy Spirit. He who serves Christ in this way is acceptable and pleasing to God and is approved by men" (AMP). The concern for acceptance from others began to diminish as Alicia's true image began to mature. The transformation had to occur from the inside first, and then make its way to the outside. Outer change without inner transformation is futile. We all need a "heart transplant" at some point in our life.

> We all need a "heart transplant" at some point in our life.

Alicia would now have the opportunity to invite the Father to make her heart His home on a daily basis. When she felt unhappy, He would comfort her. When she felt lonely, He would bring encouragement. When she felt like giving up, He would add courage and strength to continue the healthy habits she would learn. Active contentment occurs when we are moving forward and trusting God each step of the way. It's not passive or controlling. Picture a couple ballroom dancing. This is how I see our daily relationship with our heavenly Father. He is the leader and guide, and we follow. As we trust Him and allow Him to lead, the dance appears effortless and beautiful.

DIETARY CHANGES FOR OPTIMAL HEALTH

We now turned our focus on Alicia's diet and the changes she needed to make. Through analyzing her blood work, I became aware from a clinical nutrition perspective that she lacked B-complex vitamins. Symptomatically, this revealed itself as poor fat metabolism, poor muscle tone, high blood pressure, and stress syndrome. These B vitamins in particular are the lipotrophic (fat-burning) factors: choline and inositol. I gave her a supplement to support these issues. I also supported her digestive system with enzymes specific for aiding in her carbohydrate and fat metabolism. When someone is at least fifty pounds overweight, the body is supporting a great expenditure of energy, especially in the area of oxygen utilization. This oxygen debt is what causes shortness of breath and tiredness upon exertion. Alicia needed to exercise, but slowly and methodically.

We wanted her to be able to see the results of her efforts and not to have any setbacks, so we started with easy, manageable goals. She lived by a lake and found it very easy to begin walking near it every day. She also owned a treadmill. I recommended she start at an easy pace with the goal of getting her pace up to her target heart rate. To determine her target heart rate, I employed the formula found in Dr. Phil Maffetone's book *In Fitness and in Health*, called the 180-Formula.[1] According to the 180-Formula, Dr. Maffetone takes into consideration an individual's physiology and not just his or her chronological age. The 180-Formula helps an individual find his or her maximum aerobic heart rate. Instead of simply telling someone to exercise, we need to be smart and safe.

Let's figure out your 180-Formula:

1. Subtract your age from 180:
   180 − _____ (your age) = _____
2. Modify the total accordingly:
   a. Recovering from illness or surgery, subtract 10
   b. Never exercised before, subtract 5
   c. Frequently ill or have allergies, subtract 5
   d. Competitive athlete, add 5

Your final total is your maximum aerobic heart rate. If you want to enhance your aerobic capacity, exercising at this rate will accomplish your goal. The target heart range is ten beats per minute below this number. So if you have an aerobic exercise heart rate of 145, your range would be 135 to 145. It is recommended to stay within this range. It is acceptable to go below it but not above. At this point you would not feel winded and could enjoy your workout. It is said that if you can have a conversation while you walk, you are at a good pace. No matter what the sport, the target aerobic heart rate can be applied.

As Alicia began to exercise at her target heart rate, she found she was able to walk faster each week. This is when she started to notice her body fat changing. Her initial body fat composition was 38 percent. This meant that of her total weight, 38 percent of it was fat. Or in simple terms, for a 190-pound woman, 72 pounds was fat. At her ideal weight of 120 pounds, she would have no more than 25 pounds of fat.

Alicia needed to lose 70 pounds. Her goal was to lose only one pound per week and not to gain it back. This was done using a sensible eating plan.

She was accustomed to consuming large quantities of food. Instead of putting her on a calorie-restrictive diet, I allowed her to continue eating a larger than normal amount of food, but only of certain items. Alicia habitually used low-fat or nonfat salad dressings and cream products. She also drank at least three to four diet sodas per day. These had to go. Next on the list was to eliminate the bad fats in her diet. She loved French-fried potatoes. But to eliminate all the bad fats, everything fried had to go. Eventually I taught her some new ways to eat potatoes—but not fried.

For the first month we restricted carbohydrate consumption. Her diet consisted of some fruits, all vegetables, nuts, eggs, meat, fish, poultry, butter, olive oil, and flaxseed oil. For beverages, she could have herbal teas and water with lime. She could eat as much as she wanted, but only of these items. Within the first month her cholesterol dropped from 283 to 210. You may be wondering how your cholesterol can drop while you're eating fat. The way I explain it is that the body builds cholesterol not from eating cholesterol but from the amount of work it must expend to break down your foods into energy. The more processed a food is, white bread or fried potatoes for example, the more energy needed. If foods are eaten in a more natural state, the body needs less energy, and therefore the cholesterol can normalize. After the second week she could add brown rice to her dinner.

Alicia's diet could be summarized as follows:

Proteins

As much protein as desired. It is very important that a small amount of protein is consumed every two hours. It is important to buy only meats that are free of dyes, preservatives, antibiotics, and steroids. These are available at most health food markets.

Red meat—if allowed, optimally 2–3 ounces three times per week

Fish—unlimited, unbreaded

Fowl—unlimited, unbreaded

Eggs—unlimited, boiled, poached, or fried in butter or olive oil

Nuts—see Snacks

Vegetables

Steamed or raw and as fresh as possible (no canned). It is preferable to buy only organic vegetables, because they are much more nutrient rich.

Green vegetables—unlimited (e.g., chard, broccoli, spinach, zucchini, mustard and collard greens)

Yellow and orange vegetables—small portions (e.g., squash)

Fruits

All fresh fruits, allowed in the morning only. Lower carbohydrate fruits are preferred. Check out Corinne Netzer's *The Complete Book of Food Counts*[2] for actual grams. Strawberries, grapefruit, and melons are good choices.

Beverages

Ideally when thirsty, water is best with a small amount of lime. Drinking too much water can be almost as detrimental as too little. Herbal teas (no caffeine or sweetener).

Snacks

Unlimited unsalted raw nuts. Fresh fruits (morning only) and vegetables.

Grains

Brown rice may be eaten at the dinner meal only.

Oils and Spices

Flaxseed oil can be combined with raw apple cider vinegar for salad dressing. Fresh herbs for seasoning. Sea salt. Cold-pressed expeller olive oil or raw salted or unsalted butter for cooking.

Food Items Not Allowed

No wheat or wheat products, including bagels and pasta. No sugar, honey, maple syrup, etc. No hydrogenated oils. No margarine, oleo, or canola oil. No processed dairy products, except butter. (Raw dairy products are acceptable, including kefir and cottage cheese.)

This program is designed to improve the body's ability to maintain its blood sugar within a healthy range. Most of Alicia's symptoms were related to the hormonal imbalances caused by her fluctuating blood sugar. By maintaining this diet strictly, most patients see many symptoms they normally experienced dissipate. Each meal needs to contain all three major food groups: carbohydrates, proteins, and fats.

> There's no rule that says vegetables only after 11 A.M.

For breakfast, Alicia could have a two-egg omelet, cooked in butter or olive oil, with spinach, zucchini, broccoli, and mushrooms, and sliced tomatoes on the side. Another option would be two eggs scrambled with a ground turkey patty and a small salad on the side. It's okay to have non-breakfast foods at breakfast. There's no rule that says vegetables only after 11 A.M. The bigger picture was having balanced meals every time she ate. Her snacks included unsalted raw nuts and a piece of fruit or a vegetable. For lunch and dinner she could have a big salad, including a variety of vegetables with oil and vinegar or lemon dressing and a piece of grilled chicken or fish. In total, she ate three meals and two to three snacks per day. Since she didn't have to count calories, this allowed her to focus on quality and balance. It was actually fairly easy for her to do.

Alicia followed this diet for one month, having added the brown rice at the second week. She felt so good that she asked me if she could stay on it. The only consideration was that she needed to reach a point where she consumed less. We needed to make sure her meals were balanced so that as she learned what it meant to be satisfied, she could consume less food and still get her nutrients.

It takes the stomach twenty minutes to realize it is full. Most of us can consume massive quantities of food in that time. I like to encourage some basic food rules in order to gain satiation and satisfaction from our meals. In the past Alicia would inhale her food. Lesson one was to choose the place where she would eat her meals. Not on the couch or in front of the television, but at a table. Then she could create a comfortable and relaxing environment: pleasant music, mellow lighting, and maybe a scented candle. The goal was to be calm at the table so rushing the meal was less likely. As she sat to eat, she invited the Lord to join her, nourishing her mind, soul, and body as she blessed Him. She drank a full glass of water before she ate. With each bite she counted to twenty before swallowing. I wanted her to slow down and develop a sense of what foods really tasted like. When people overeat, they tend not to chew or even taste the food.

I once taught a nutrition seminar at a school for the blind. I had the students taste various foods, smell them, and feel them, noticing the texture and shape. It was a wonderful "sense-perience" that opened their inner eyes to foods in a different way. I shared this with Alicia. She soon appreciated the smell and taste of foods. As she began to eat slower, chew her foods, and experience less stress at each meal, she felt full faster, and over time was able to eat less. Numerous studies link overindulging with heart and other degenerative diseases. The habit of eating less has benefits beyond weight loss.

As the months passed, Alicia stuck to her diet. Eventually we sparingly added some whole grains and potatoes. I taught her how to make oven-baked French fries by cutting the potato or yam and baking the pieces on a cookie sheet with a small amount of olive oil, sea salt, pepper, and various herbs that she liked. It

> ## Numerous studies link overindulging with heart and other degenerative diseases.

hit the spot. To substitute her ice-cream craving, she froze bananas and blended them with a few unsalted nuts. For Alicia, this was a home run.

Over a period of a year and a half, Alicia lost her weight and kept it off. She not only became healthy physically but spiritually as well. Her life was absolutely transformed by coming to a true knowledge of the Father and seeing how trapped she had been living. She wants to become a nutritionist and is now studying to do so. I am proud to have been used by God in her transformation.

Maybe you saw some similarities between Alicia's life and your own. Has bitterness stopped you from entering into God's presence? Have you been paying a debt from your childhood by holding onto that extra weight? If so, pray with me that freedom may come as the Sun of Righteousness arises with healing in His wings.

Father, I know there are many who hope yet live daily having their needs only temporarily met, not by you but by the world. I know there is true freedom available in you. I ask you to lift us up from the steps of our existence, strengthen feeble knees, and allow us to see what you have for us. Help us to trust you to meet all our needs as a mother meets her baby's needs. Help us not to rebel but to yield and surrender our all to you.

But unto you who revere and worshipfully fear My name shall the Sun of Righteousness arise with healing in His wings.

MALACHI 4:2 AMP

FIT TIP #26:

Exercise at or below your target heart rate for maximum aerobic efficiency. Use the 180-Formula to determine your maximum aerobic target heart rate.

FIT TIP #27:

Determine where you will eat your meals and create a healing environment for your senses. Play soothing music, have pleasant lighting, light scented candles. Use the "good" dishes and enjoy every aspect of every meal.

FIT TIP #28:

Count to twenty after each bite. Remember, it takes twenty minutes for your brain to notice your stomach is full. Take your time and relax.

10
FREE TO BE FIT

A Purpose for Living

I met Doris at a community health fair. Impeccably dressed, with her matching scarf neatly disguising her aging neck, she was graceful and sporty, meandering through the various health-care booths. When she approached my booth, I found her charming and beautiful. A woman in her late sixties, she felt that life was basically over, yet she longed to feel young once again. Her children had their lives, and her husband had passed away five years prior. She wanted solutions for her weight, her achy joints, and her seemingly daily atrophying muscles and strength. She and her husband had played tennis together, snow skied, camped, and hiked, as well as participated in numerous athletic events. Now she felt old, and many of her friends had already given in to senior living. I suggested we get together for a consultation so I could get to know her better and find out what was really going on with her health.

We met the following week. She had a look of anticipation and excitement on her face and joyfully announced, "I just know you can help me. This is an answer to prayer." Because she didn't yet fully understand what type of practice

I had, I hoped she would not have such high expectations that they would be humanly impossible to meet. I call this the "Cinderella" phenomenon. Sometimes patients come in with the expectation that a doctor can wave a magic wand over them, and—*poof!*—they are thin, healed, and energized. I neither carry magic dust nor a long, glittery wand. I simply care for my patients and try to offer sound, time-tested advice that will help the body be all it was designed to be. I educate my patients as well as provide clinical nutritional support for various health challenges. I wanted Doris to have a realistic yet optimistic attitude of what we could accomplish together.

As part of my general assessment of new patients, in addition to my evaluation, I have them keep a diet diary. We also discuss their goals, dreams, and fears, and try to prioritize what our plan of action will be. What was really on this dear sister's heart? What did she really want from me, and more important, what did she want from God and from herself? My role is to support those goals rather than to impose my goals.

> It was hard for Doris to believe that God still had a purpose for her life.

Doris felt as though time had somehow swept her away, and one day she woke up "old." After her husband's death, she went through such a long period of grieving that she really did believe all hope was lost, and her remaining days on earth would be simply waiting for the Lord to take her home. It was hard for Doris to believe that God still had a purpose for her life. I believed that if she could just get hold of the garment of His precious promises for her, she could possess the resurrection power of Jesus Christ. Prayerfully we asked the Lord to give Doris eyes to see herself as He saw her and to show us the specific areas we needed to address.

As with the woman in the Gospels who had the issue of blood, Doris needed a focused intensity that said, "If there is a way, it's this way. If I can just touch the hem of His garment, I know I will be made whole." Doris needed to know where her strength came from. For years she had relied on her husband for strength. Now she was on her own, trying to figure out this rapidly changing world without him.

She lacked energy as well as mental clarity; physically, she had an extra forty pounds on her petite frame and needed to build muscle strength. All the weight lingered around her hips and thighs, while her arms and upper body appeared limp, like a plant that hadn't been watered in a while. She jokingly said her waistline measured only 21 inches when she got married and now she felt more like her IQ was approaching 21. But God is gracious to us as we diligently seek Him, even for our health and life enhancement. Doris's attitude had her living with one foot in the grave and the other on a banana peel. God's intention was that she confidently put one foot in front of the other, trusting Him daily to reveal His plan for this winter season of her life. And He would prove himself to be faithful.

Doris reminded me of Sarah in the Bible, as I encouraged her that it was possible to have strength, energy, and a healthier body. She laughed as though in disbelief. But as God assured Sarah, He assured Doris as He does all of us to believe Him for impossible things. "Therefore Sarah laughed within herself, saying, 'After I have grown old, shall I have pleasure, my lord being old also?' And the Lord said to Abraham, 'Why did Sarah laugh, saying, "Shall I surely bear a child, since I am old?'" Is anything too hard for the Lord?'" (Genesis 18:12–14).

Nothing is too hard for God, but when our present circumstance and our past scream louder than our faith, it's easy to laugh in unbelief. If we look through Scripture, we will find this to be the primary request of the Father: *believe.* Belief brings about the motivation to take action, whether the action is changing our diet or spending time in prayer. I think the real root behind unbelief is fear. We are afraid that God really doesn't care about our day-in and day-out issues. We are afraid to believe, in case it doesn't work. It's easier to believe in nothing; then if nothing happens, we're not disappointed. In verse 15, Sarah denied laughing because she was afraid. Perhaps it was easier to deny her unbelief than to admit she was really afraid to trust God for an impossible thing.

How does this apply to weight loss or health improvement? If we can believe that He can and will do "exceeding abundantly above all that we ask or think" (Ephesians 3:20), we can trust Him to lead us in feeling good about ourselves, acquiring more energy, or losing a few pounds. The Father cares about it *all.* Many saints, including Doris, do not connect their spiritual life with their physical and emotional life. Doris saw them as separate entities. She prayed and went to church, but never thought about seeking God for all she needed in this season of her life. But He was calling her to a deeper level of faith.

After Doris and I discussed her history, her goals and fears were laid out on the table. She had also mentioned that she recently had a bone density test with poor results and felt her only hope to avoid osteoporosis was medication. My evaluation revealed several interesting findings. She was not digesting her food, her tissues were not absorbing minerals properly, and her saliva pH was extremely acidic. Our plan was simple and straightforward, and with the commitment to stay focused and disciplined, almost foolproof.

SOLVING, NOT MASKING, DIGESTIVE PROBLEMS

Doris had taken antacids for nearly half her life. She had become so reliant on them that she chewed them after every meal. Unfortunately, Doris did not have an excess of acid but rather a deficiency. Since her saliva pH was so acidic, Doris's stomach couldn't produce the acid it needed to properly digest her food. This may seem like a contradiction, but it's true. It is organic acid that causes indigestion and bloating after eating, not too much acid. Her meals would remain in her stomach and putrefy, making her bloat and feel very uncomfortable. Our goal was to help her stomach produce acid properly, and not merely remove the symptoms of poor digestion by neutralizing the acids.

> The calcium in antacids is not the type that supports healthy bone development.

I gave her a supplement that contained okra pepsin and hydrochloric acid as well as some wonderful proteolytic (protein digesting) digestive enzymes. She was to take them at each meal with a tall glass of room-temperature water. I also suggested she give her little "rolls of relief" a rest to see if this new plan was working for her. After about a month she noticed her bloating was drastically reduced. She wondered about her calcium intake, since her antacids also supplied her with calcium. Unfortunately, the calcium in antacids is not the type that supports healthy bone development, so I recommended a calcium-magnesium supplement. This would support her calcium need and was easily absorbed and digested. Many patients suffer with indigestion. The technical term is achlorhydria, or lack of hydrochloric acid. But because Doris had suffered with this problem for so many years, she was also unable to absorb the minerals from her food. This, in addition to being raised on and presently living on canned foods, contributed to her poor bone density score.

Clinically, I have observed that most if not all patients with weight issues also have some sort of digestive or assimilation problem. So many people want something to speed up their metabolism, when what is really needed is a clear look at the foundations of their health: the most important foundation being digestion. The body cannot function well when nutrients are not properly absorbed and toxins are not properly eliminated. Imagine a city where trash cans are spilling over into the streets, but the roads are blocked so that the trash collectors are unable to get in to empty them. Eventually rats and other pestilence overtake the city. This is how our bodies are functioning when we have poor digestion. Just because someone does not develop gas and bloating doesn't mean she has an efficient digestive system. There are other components to digestion as well.

From the mouth to the colon, there are hundreds of functions that contribute to overall health. But one fact cannot be denied; when the saliva pH is too acidic, it is impossible to have proper digestion. It is not necessary to focus on anything below the mouth if that one factor is not corrected. To make the saliva alkaline is not that difficult, but it does take some effort. More than any other contributing factor to an acidic saliva pH is the consumption of white sugar and high amounts of red meats. Sugar is the worse of the two.

Like many, Doris admitted her daily sugar indulgence. She told me she wanted a little sweetness after dinner to satisfy her. But she didn't realize, as most don't, that refined sugar is not a food but a destructive drug. It has zero nutritional value. Just a "spoonful of sugar" does not make the medicine go down any bet-

> Just a "spoonful of sugar" does not make the medicine go down any better.

ter. The human digestive tract was never intended to handle refined sugar, and it never will. Sugar causes a host of imbalances. *Lick the Sugar Habit*, by Nancy Appleton, Ph.D., offers probably the most definitive list of the damaging effects of sugar.[1] Here are just a few:

> Refined sugar can suppress the immune system; upset the body's mineral balance; cause hyperactivity, anxiety, concentration difficulties, and crankiness in children; cause drowsiness and decreased activity in children; adversely affect children's school grades; produce a significant rise in triglycerides; contribute to a weakened defense against bacterial infection; cause kidney damage; reduce helpful high-density lipoproteins (HDLs); promote an elevation of harmful low-density lipoproteins (LDLs); lead to chromium deficiency; cause copper deficiency; interfere with the absorption of calcium and magnesium; lead to breast, ovarian, prostate, and rectal cancer; cause colon cancer, with an increased risk in women; be a risk factor in gallbladder cancer; increase fasting levels of

glucose; weaken eyesight; raise the level of a neurotransmitter called serotonin, which can narrow blood vessels; cause hypoglycemia; produce an acidic saliva; raise adrenaline levels in children; malabsorption is common in those with functional bowel disease; speed the aging process, causing wrinkles and gray hair; lead to alcoholism; promote tooth decay; contribute to weight gain and obesity; [high intake] increases the risk of Crohn's disease and ulcerative colitis; cause a raw inflamed intestinal tract in persons with gastric or duodenal ulcers; cause arthritis; asthma; candidiasis (yeast infection); lead to the formation of gallstones; lead to the formation of kidney stones; cause ischemic heart disease; cause appendicitis; exacerbate the symptoms of multiple sclerosis; indirectly cause hemorrhoids; cause varicose veins; elevate glucose and insulin responses in oral contraceptive users; lead to periodontal disease; contribute to osteoporosis; contribute to saliva activity; cause a decrease in insulin sensitivity; lead to decreased glucose tolerance; decrease growth hormone; increase cholesterol; increase systolic blood pressure; change the structure of protein, causing interference with protein absorption; cause food allergies; contribute to diabetes; cause toxemia during pregnancy; contribute to eczema in children; cause cardiovascular disease; impair the structure of DNA; cause cataracts; cause emphysema; cause arteriosclerosis; cause free-radical formation in the bloodstream; lower the enzymes' ability to function; cause loss of tissue elasticity and function; cause liver cells to divide, increasing the size of the liver; increase the amount of fat in the liver; increase kidney size and produce pathological changes in the kidney; overstress the pancreas, causing damage; increase the body's fluid retention; cause constipation; cause myopia (nearsightedness); compromise the lining of the capillaries; cause tendons to become brittle; cause headaches, including migraines; cause an increase in delta, alpha, and theta brain waves, which can alter the ability to think clearly; cause depression; increase insulin responses in those consuming high-sugar diets compared to low-sugar diets; increase bacterial fermentation in the colon; cause hormonal imbalance; cause blood platelet adhesiveness, which causes blood clots.

Overwhelming, isn't it? I often print this list out and give it to patients who wonder, "Is it really that bad?" YES! I had Doris put the printout on her refrigerator and highlight the specific issues she was dealing with. Whenever she was tempted to satisfy that little craving, she would read the highlighted items. Sometimes it worked and other times the present temptation had a greater impact on her than the possibility of a future problem. Of course, the next logical question was, "What about artificial sweeteners?" Much worse. According to historical nutrition researcher and dentist Dr. Melvin Page, "When a person has been accustomed to artificial sweeteners and refined sugars, it usually takes about three to four weeks for him to regain his natural taste for sweetness after having dispensed with the use of these drugs and/or sugar."[2] There are products that can help the body restore a normal pH, but the elimination of refined sugar and artificial sweeteners is the best way to accomplish this. The principle is "God-made is always better than man-made."

I assured Doris that eventually her sugar cravings would subside and healthy sugars, such as fresh fruit, would taste great when her taste buds were healed. Since she had been accustomed to canned fruits and artificial sweeteners, fresh fruit tasted unnatural. She had a false sense of sweetness that had dulled her sensitivity to natural sweetness. Eventually Doris was free from her antacids and her sugar. As her digestion improved, she noticed that her appetite also started to decrease. I recommended she eat several small meals per day; each should include vegetables, no more than three ounces of hormone-free animal protein, and a small amount of whole grain. Protein requirements should be increased in seniors, as this may help reduce the risk of bone loss and has been associated with declines in loss of muscle mass as well as a decrease in fracture rate. However, too much protein can lead to bone loss.[3]

SLOW AND STEADY WEIGHT LOSS

Doris lost forty pounds in about one year. Slowly, healthily, and methodically, the pounds came off. Doris's program also included exercise. Light weight lifting and mild, consistent cardiovascular exercise helps to improve bone density. Doris joined the local women's gym and took a cardio-strength training class three times per week. She power-walked two days a week with a woman from her church, who was also a widow. They made a commitment to pray when they walked. In fact, they became not only prayer partners but fitness accountability partners as well.

This season in her life was one of discovery, although she still had some fears. Yet as she focused on Jesus, He began to reveal himself to her in ways that were most amazing. God gave a specific promise to Doris and her walking partner: "Fear not, for you shall not be ashamed; neither be confounded and depressed, for you shall not be put to shame; for you shall forget the shame of your youth, and you shall not [seriously] remember the reproach of your widowhood any more. For your Maker is your husband, the Lord of hosts is His name; and the

Holy One of Israel is your Redeemer; the God of the whole earth He is called" (Isaiah 54:4–5 AMP).

The Lord did indeed have a plan for Doris's winter season; He wasn't about to let her slip into oblivion, thinking her life was over because her earthly love was no longer with her. God blessed her with such compassion. She was probably the best listener I have ever met. It seemed like the Spirit of God spoke through her when she gave comfort to those who were hurting. This is truly a gift from God to humanity. An opportunity presented itself at a Christian shelter for battered, abused, and drug-addicted women. Doris began to go there weekly and offer aid in whatever way she could. She found herself one on one with at least one woman per week, just listening. Little by little, Doris's presence at the shelter became a light as she brought words of hope and encouragement to these seemingly hopeless women. Doris was blessed and finally began to see the purpose of this time in her life. She pressed in, powered up, and is now powering out by helping others.

Perhaps you have entered a season of uncertainty, filled with change and confusion. Let me pray with you that you will come to know God's purpose during this time.

Father, in the name of Jesus, your Word assures us that you indeed have a plan and purpose for our lives and that it is good. Though we can't always see it, and the way is rarely clear, we can feel secure that because you are sovereign we can trust you. Fill us afresh today with confidence, clarity, and the desire to persistently seek your face no matter what we see, feel, or believe. Give us eyes to see the needs of others and the compassion to take action. And while we turn our eyes off of ourselves, give us the faith that you will meet our needs. Amen.

For this is what the Lord says: "I will extend peace to her like a river, and the wealth of nations like a flooding stream; you will nurse and be carried on her arm and dandled on her knees. As a mother comforts her child, so will I comfort you; and you will be comforted over Jerusalem."

ISAIAH 66:12–13 NIV

FIT TIP #29:

Quit eating refined sugar. It's not good for you; you do know that by now, don't you?

FIT TIP #30:

Light weight lifting and mild cardiovascular exercise at least three times a week for no less than twenty minutes each time can help support and strengthen bone density. Speak to your physician and consult a personal trainer at the gym for exercises and limitations.

FIT TIP #31:

Develop an impulse strategy. When you crave sweets, know ahead of time what you will do about it. Whatever your vulnerable issue is, decide beforehand how you will manage it and tell your fitness accountability partner for added support.

FIT TIP #32:

Eat foods that are God-made. Buy fresh produce instead of canned. Canned foods have preservatives that are not conducive to life and health.

11

FIT FIGHT

Learning to Say No

Janine knew the call God had on her life. She was a pastor's kid with a burden to pray for others ever since she could remember. Now a pastor's wife and in charge of the intercessory prayer group in her church, she was confident that she was where God wanted her to be. Janine was the dutiful daughter, the dutiful wife, and the dutiful mother. Compelled to always do the right thing, she found it difficult to say no. After all, it is godly to serve, isn't it? Consequently, she rarely, if ever, said no to anyone about anything, until it began to wear her out.

Janine had such a love and compassion for people that she never realized her lack of healthy boundaries and self-care had taken a toll on her hormone balance and her metabolism. She was typically tired and—more often than she liked to admit—cranky. But she always greeted her family, friends, and congregation members with a smile rather than any hint of what she was really feeling. She began to question her motivation. Was she serving out of fear of what people would think if she did say no, or because she was a nice person—who now needed to set some personal boundaries if she was going to be of any help to anyone.

Between the bake sales, attendance at food-laden conferences, late-night dinners, and simply not having the time to take care of herself, Janine was becoming increasingly aware of how uncomfortable she felt: insignificant, unattractive, and vaguely sick. Janine also was beginning to feel intimidated by the more "attractive" women in her church. Her husband repeatedly told her how beautiful she was, but she had a tough time receiving his kind and sincere compliments. Unfortunately, Janine had started to believe the lies she heard in her head as she looked in the mirror: *Janine, you are fat, and no one will ever respect you, listen to you, or think you're pretty.*

A young woman in their church started teaching aerobics and encouraged Janine to attend, but Janine couldn't imagine wearing exercise clothes and lining up next to the "attractive" women in the church. She did attend one class, but the well-meaning instructor wanted to help everyone set some healthy goals, so she had the women weigh in. (When someone is extremely pound conscious, I prefer having her measure herself with a tape measure so the focus is not on "the weight number.") When Janine saw that she weighed thirty pounds more than she did before her children were born, she was horrified. She knew her weight had crept up on her, but she didn't think it was that much. She wore loose-fitting clothing most of the time, so couldn't gauge her weight by how they fit. Now that she knew "the number" she was completely mortified and could think about nothing else. She didn't want aerobics; she wanted a miracle.

She appeared ashamed as she sat in my office, expressing her guilt over her weight gain. She accepted full responsibility but was completely immobilized by this revelation. On the verge of tears, she was desperate:

> She didn't want aerobics; she wanted a miracle.

"I'll do whatever I need to do to lose weight." There was no quick, healthy solution to her challenge.

"I'm only forty-seven years old. I'm not supposed to be fat yet," she sighed. She equated weight gain with the aging process. Many people ascribe to this belief. It's true that certain hormonal changes affect metabolic functions, but this is not only because of age. Many mature adults have learned how to eat well and live with a healthy balanced weight. Janine said that her mom was noticeably overweight in her forties, and now she feared the same was in store for her. She looked at her thighs as if they were an enemy, and in absolute anguish she moaned, "My mom has really bad cellulite, and look, I'm getting it too!"

As a culture we are getting sicker while our waists are expanding. The statistics for obesity, heart disease, and other degenerative diseases are on the rise. One would think that with so many diets available, we would be able to follow one and lose weight permanently. We seem to be fencing against an invisible enemy, but not the right one. Ephesians 6:12 tells us that we aren't fighting against flesh and blood but against spiritual forces. Yet in our battle with the bulge, we find ourselves fighting ourselves and our own fleshly desires. It seems to me that if we could deal with our aberrant thoughts and habits, we could focus our energy and attention on the real enemy: the Enemy of our souls and Accuser of the brethren. As long as Satan can keep our attention fixed on our desolate waist, he knows we won't focus our attention in the areas that really matter to the kingdom of God, the desolate wasteland of barren souls.

How does one make the transition from such an earthly focus to a godly one? How could Janine change her focus from her thighs to being that powerful intercessor she was called to be? It came down to acknowledging that her focus was off. She had indulged her appetite for such a long time that her weight had crept up on her. She was so busy doing God's work that she forgot about taking care of her temple, daily remaining sober and vigilant. While she wanted to wage war against her widening waistline, she needed to first acknowledge that she had violated her body with junk foods over a period of many years.

We are given treasures in earthen vessels, but sometimes we forget that the vessel is a gift from God that must be taken care of. After all, it has to last us a long time. Sometimes we expect too much from our body. We expect it to be able to turn junk into nutrition when we eat nutrient-starved foods. But then we get frustrated when we gain weight or our cholesterol is too high. The truth you know will set you free. I believe God gives us grace in the areas where we lack knowledge. But once we have knowledge, we are responsible to abide by it. God's grace will meet us to the degree we have been taught the truth.

HORMONAL CHANGES AT MID-LIFE

Janine was pre-menopausal. In addition to her weight gain, she also noticed that she was extremely emotional. She found herself crying at the most ridiculous things. She battled with what she called "seasonal" allergies and constipation. Her menstrual cycles were beginning to become irregular, and she was starting to have hot flashes, fatigue, insomnia, headaches, and anxiety. She didn't want to admit it, but her sex drive had plummeted to an all-time low. Among the possibilities that could be causing her weight gain and various other symptoms, the first consideration was to look at her hormones.

We did a salivary female hormone profile taken over an eleven-day period. This test showed us her estrogen, progesterone, and testosterone levels, as well as other adrenal hormones. As it turned out, she was beginning menopause, and much of what she was feeling emotionally was due to the hormonal changes she was experiencing. This didn't make our goal any easier. When a woman begins menopause, it is a time of great transition. This is not a time to *get* healthy but to harness the resources of years of taking care of oneself so that the ammunition is available to keep the ship sailing smoothly. But if diet and stress levels have depleted those reserves, menopause will be a difficult road to travel. Fortunately, with God nothing is impossible.

Janine, like many women, was unaware that menopause was not an end but a transition to a new season of life. She had a lot of fear involved in this "change of life." *Will I still be feminine? Will I grow facial hair? Will I still have my sexuality?* These are but a few of the questions that ran through her mind. As the estrogen begins to decline over a period of years, unless induced by surgery or chemotherapy, the changes also occur over several years. The adrenal glands, or stress-fighting glands, pick up the slack by producing a certain amount of an androgen hormone that is converted into estrogen, if they are functioning properly. But if they are depleted through chronic stress and poor diet, the estrogen production is compromised.

Janine reviewed her test results with her medical doctor to weigh her options of natural or chemical hormone-replacement therapy. The three of us decided to begin with natural progesterone, natural support to increase her testosterone levels, a liver and bowel detoxification program, and, of course, some major dietary changes.

I would like to add a warning at this point. Another patient asked me to bring some clarity to a mail-order lab test she had performed because her progesterone and testosterone levels seemed off the charts. She wondered if she was reading the test incorrectly. I phoned the lab, and her hormones were indeed off the charts. She had been using an over-the-counter cream containing wild yam and other "natural" ingredients that support an increase in progesterone, but it had extremely detrimental effects on her total female hormone profile. The lab instructed her to discontinue use of this product. I'm sharing this not to frighten you, but to protect you from taking your health into your own hands and self-medicating with things that *seem* healthy. There is a natural synergy that all nutrients and medications should have. Even if something is "natural," it does not mean it is right for you or that it will support your total health restoration program.

Always consult your physician before taking any—even natural—substances. I think it is a good idea to have two doctors: your medical physician and your natural care physician. Optimally it would be wonderful if they could consult with each other regarding your care to ensure your total health needs are considered and supported. This worked well for Janine, and if your doctor is willing, it may work well for you.

Janine's diet consisted of just about everything unhealthy, and she had no idea that it had thrown her hormones off balance. We knew from the tests that Janine's adrenals were also stressed. Goodies like caffeine, bad fats, white flour, sugar, and basically any processed foods cause unnecessary stress to the adrenals. Of course, emotional stress contributes to this more than any foods can. As Janine had been pouring her life out in service, she hadn't been replenishing it with nourishment, and now she was paying the price.

> The liver's main responsibility is to break down the chemicals that we take in from the environment.

The adrenals are not alone in this fight. The entire alliance of hormone-producing glands works together, along with the body's garbage disposal, the liver, to help keep our body in balance. The liver is the largest organ in the body and has a huge role in the processing of nutrients. In addition to processing fats, carbohydrates, and proteins, it filters toxins, including bacteria and allergens, from the blood. It also detoxifies toxic chemicals and natural toxins such as mold and fungi, hormones, histamines, and ammonia. The liver's main responsibility is to break down the chemicals that we take in from the environment. Since the liver is the entry to the body, it is easy to see how it can get overloaded. In one day we can encounter over seven hundred foreign chemicals, from dry-cleaning fluid and copier toner to chemicals on new linens, pesticides, air pollutants, and additives to our foods and drinks. The liver has a huge job.

When we are young, our liver is able to detoxify most of the destructive things we do to it without any difficulty. But as we grow older, its detoxifying capacity wanes, and we begin to exhibit the symptoms of liver stress. Many people simply cover the symptoms of liver stress with an over-the-counter remedy: caffeine for the fatigue, Tylenol for the headache, Ex-Lax for the constipation, Allegra for the allergies, etc. All are mere Band-Aids on an underlying imbalance. If the liver is toxic, as is the case for most people in a civilized society eating the typical diet, then it is very likely that hormonal as well as other imbalances exist. This was Janine's situation.

Janine was more than willing to start the process of living a balanced life. On each level she made commitments to regain her true purpose and function healthily. On the nutritional level, we decided to begin with a liver and gastro-intestinal detoxification program to repair the damage her diet had caused. A healthy liver and gastrointestinal program should be monitored by a physician. I recommend whole-food nutrients, herbs, and homeopathic remedies. The process is so individual that it is difficult to offer general suggestions. What was used in Janine's case may not be the best recommendation in your situation. *Do not self-medicate.* For some patients the process is very simple, while for others there may be the need to proceed slowly and use very gentle products.

To help her gastrointestinal system start working better, Janine was given Zypan[1] and UltraClear medical food[2] to take for one month along with digestive enzymes. This combination would help strengthen and detoxify her liver and gastrointestinal system. I gave her plenty of antioxidants[3], organic minerals, and trace minerals to support the entire process and help the liver recover from the oxidative stress of life in a civilized country.

A four-part plan

The entire program consisted of four parts:

1. REMOVE or eliminate any unhealthy foods and sources of stress from the diet.
2. REPLACE with healthy sources of nutrition.
3. REPAIR the liver and digestive system.
4. REDUCE emotional stress and focus on improving stress management.

Step one was the REMOVAL of the toxins and dietary factors that were causing stress to her system. The worst are hydrogenated and partially hydrogenated fats. Many fad diets tell you to eat a low-fat or nonfat diet. I recall a certain infomercial that said you could lose weight by counting your fat grams. You can, but will you be any healthier? Fat is essential for health. It's the bad fats that we need to eliminate. That's why there are substances called essential fatty acids—because they are *essential*. When essential fats are missing, several problems arise, including female hormone and menstrual irregularities, such as PMS, scanty or missed periods, cramps, and skin problems, plus problems such as headaches, joint pain, asthma, and hot flashes. To worsen an already dismal situation, these essential fats are often replaced with rancid, synthetic fats that are actually poisons. The highly processed fats and oils do not supply the body with the needed nutrition.

This is an alert. Remove these items from your kitchen: hydrogenated fats or oils or partially hydrogenated fats or oils. They are poison. Check your labels and you'll see they are in everything from salad dressings, margarines, and shortenings to nondairy creamers and nondairy milk products, such as cocoa mixes and sauces.

Hydrogenated fats or oils and partially hydrogenated fats or oils do not exist in nature. These fats are extremely toxic to the human body. They are processed as they are for the sole purpose of lengthening the product's shelf life, not your life. They are also called "trans" fats because they are manipulated in the laboratory in such a way that when you eat them they are incorporated into your cell membranes, altering the configuration of these delicate structures. Hydrogenated fats or oils and partially hydrogenated fats or oils inhibit the body's normal metabolism of fats and stay in the body on an average of fifty-one days before they are totally metabolized.

Healthy fats in the diet produce hormones called prostaglandins (PGs). Several essential functions in the body rely on these PGs. There are good PGs and bad PGs. The bad ones are the culprits for many connective tissue diseases (heart disease, stroke, cancer, and autoimmune diseases, for example) in our society. They are found in red meats, shellfish, and dairy products. These items are high in what are called omega-6 fatty acids. Though they produce some good PGs, two-thirds are converted to the pro-inflammatory hormone form. On the other hand, the good PGs counteract the negative effects of the bad PGs. Simply put, trans fats block the production of good PGs, and by default the bad PGs are produced without hindrance.

In addition to trans fats facilitating the increase of bad PG production, other substances also inhibit good PG production, including aspirin, acetaminophen, and other non-steroidal anti-inflammatories (NSAIDs), such as ibuprofen and naproxen, typically taken to alleviate the symptoms of bad PG abuse (headaches, joint pain, PMS). These drugs work by inhibiting good PG production.

Next, we remove fried foods and fatty meat products. The chemicals, hormones, and steroids used in preserving meats are stored in the fatty tissues of the animal. As we consume these items we also consume the chemicals.

THE "GRACE DIET"

What to do? First, stop eating trans fats that provide absolutely no nutrition. Next, REPLACE these bad fats with high-quality good fat to repair and protect your body. Foods that contain good fats are raw unsalted nuts, avocados, and raw flaxseed oil (cold use only). Eat meats that are hormone-, antibiotic-, and chemical-free. If these are not available, choose lean meats and better cuts of meat. The fats naturally found in fish are a great source of essential fatty acids. The cold-water fish are especially beneficial, including salmon, herring, mackerel, and sardines. Olive oil and butter in moderation are also excellent healthy omega-6 fat sources, and are especially useful for cooking. You'll find healthy oils (olive and flaxseed) in the refrigerated section of the health food market.

If you are already having health problems from years of consuming bad fats, I recommend three specific nutritional compounds: (1) a good source of vitamins A, C, P, and bioflavonoids. These are excellent antioxidants. (2) a female protomorphogen product containing extracts of the female reproductive gland and/or organs[4] and a good source of raw chlorophyll that contains more fat-soluble nutrition, which are additional female hormone precursors.[5] (3) an excellent source of omega-3 and omega-6 fatty acids, such as found in flaxseed oil, borage oil, and black currant seed oil. Realistically, it will take six to nine months to restore the damage done by bad fats in your system. But most people notice an improvement in a much shorter time than that.

Although I would have liked to have seen Janine convert her kitchen overnight to a totally organic, raw food haven, I knew this would not happen. Instead, I taught her, as I do all my patients, that the gradual "grace diet" was the best way to go. In the "grace diet" we go from bad, to better, to best as we can comfortably and reasonably make the changes. For some, this process may take many years.

> In the "grace diet" we go from bad, to better, to best as we can comfortably and reasonably make the changes.

The "grace diet" is a gradual process that has been one of the most helpful tools for women who want to feed their family healthier foods without creating a war in their home. It is a way to begin substituting healthier items one by one in such a way that the family hardly realizes you are doing it. For example, instead of having sodas in the refrigerator, make homemade lemonade or iced tea, or make homemade macaroni and cheese instead of using a prepared boxed mix. Another suggestion is to focus for a three-month period on reducing or eliminating refined sugar from the family diet. These are examples of going from bad to better.

Each person has his or her bad, better, and best program. I suggest patients highlight in their diet diaries what they think is really bad, not so bad, and good. This lets me know what they are thinking. If a patient thinks canned fruit is a healthy food, we start there. I would encourage this person to eat fresh fruit instead. To some, this sounds obvious, but to others, canned foods are a way of life.

After we remove the bad fats from our diet, we turn our focus to carbohydrates. Carbohydrates are found in fruits, vegetables, breads, starches, baked goods, and grain products. In and of themselves, carbohydrates are not bad. It's what is done to them between their natural state and their appearance on our plates that determines whether or not they are bad for us. Other determining factors are how we prepare them, how much of them we eat, and with what other foods we eat them. Many people are confused over the carbohydrate issue.

Bad carbohydrates are white bread, processed wheat bread, white pasta, standard store-bought muffins, cakes, and cookies, boxed rice or potato mixes, and white rice. When a grain is enriched—to prolong shelf life—most of the nutrition is destroyed and a few synthetic factors are added back. I don't know about you, but when someone takes more than thirty vital ingredients away and adds back four synthetic factors, I don't feel enriched. Needless to say, this process is damaging to our health; all enriched grain products should be avoided.

As far as other carbohydrates are concerned, always keep in mind that fresh is best. By eating canned or packaged foods, you are losing much of the vital nutrition. Even when cooked properly, foods lose their nutritive value if not eaten promptly. The fresher the foods the more nutrient-dense they are. Steaming vegetables or eating them raw is a wonderful way to preserve the nutrients found in them. I often recommend purchasing vegetarian cookbooks to get ideas on creative ways to prepare vegetables. Moderation is equally important. I usually recommend to my patients that they eat small portions of grains and starches so they won't have blood sugar problems. Eating a large plate of spaghetti puts a lot of strain on the pancreas. But if a smaller helping of spaghetti is eaten with a small amount of meat, a salad, and lots of steamed or raw vegetables, it's not so bad. By replacing the processed carbohydrates with fresh, nutrient-rich sources in moderation, it is easy to trim some extra pounds and become healthier. While many claim that counting calories is the key to permanent weight loss, I have found that a diet high in nutrient-dense foods eaten frequently and in moderation precludes the necessity to count calories.

The "better" alternatives to enriched bread and grain products are the organic, whole, or sprouted grain products available in health food stores. Choosing brown or wild rice instead of white rice is a "better" choice. Anything steamed or baked over anything fried is a "better" choice. The "best" alternative for bread is to purchase a grain mill and make your own bread.

The third food group to remove from the diet is processed dairy products. I believe that our Creator knew what He was doing when He made the items He recommended we eat. Everything God-made is in perfect balance and synergy. When man starts altering the food supply with his limited knowledge, problems occur. Most people are not able to find raw dairy products because the government has placed tremendous restrictions on them. But they are the best source of nutrition from dairy.

I recommend having no dairy products at all rather than consuming dairy that is pasteurized and homogenized. My primary concern with pasteurization is that it destroys most of the needed vitamins and enzymes at the same time that it kills unwanted bacteria. There are other sources of calcium that are better. For more about processed and raw dairy products see Appendix B.

For raw milk, cows must be healthier to start with. They are not given drugs to pretty them up or steroids to fatten them. Overall, the entire certified raw milk process is a cleaner, healthier one. Yet we are told that raw milk is dangerous. God placed within our bodies the immune system. This alliance of organs and processes is designed to alert us of unwanted organisms and effectively deal with them. Bacteria are not the enemy. Denatured and adulterated foods are the enemy. Our bodies know what to do with bacteria, but they cannot deal with a denatured food. The body recognizes an item as either a food or a toxin. The body cannot recognize pasteurized, homogenized, and fortified milk as a food, and uses various means to rid the body of it. Numerous studies have linked pasteurized milk with breast cancer and other bowel-related cancers.[6] What I have observed is that people with dairy allergies or lactose intolerance tend not to have these sensitivities while on raw dairy products. The enzymes present in raw milk aid the body in digesting the milk. This lessens the stress on the pancreas.

The "best" alternative in the dairy arena is raw. I would say that none is the "better" choice if raw throws you into shock or if it's not available. Green leafy vegetables, kiwi, and cantaloupe all have rich sources of many of the same nutrients found in milk products and are excellent replacements. Further, I believe nonfat and low-fat milk products should be avoided even more than whole milk. The balance has been so altered by reducing the fat that the sugar content is too high for the pancreas to handle. Imagine fat as the clutch and the milk sugar as the accelerator. The clutch helps to control the acceleration. Keep this in mind with any nonfat or low-fat food product.

Let's take a look at soy. Soybeans are an excellent source of protein and they are a good source of natural plant estrogens called phytoestrogens. Phytoestrogens are known to have wonderful immune-strengthening properties. So don't be afraid of tofu. There are many delicious recipes for tofu. I have made tofu enchiladas that tasted very much like chicken. It's all in the seasoning, because tofu doesn't have any taste in itself. The only good soy products are the natural, unadulterated forms like tofu, miso, and steamed soybeans. Now for the bad news. Commercial renditions of healthy soy products border on blasphemy. Commercial producers tell us that soy ice cream or soy hot dogs are a good source of the nutrients contained in natural soy. Not so. For information on the dangers of soy, take a look at the Weston A. Price Foundation Web site: *www.westonaprice.org*. An article called "Soy Alert" is quite informative.

What healthy beverages can you drink to replace fruit juices, sodas, coffee, and alcohol? Fruit is meant to be eaten whole, not drunk as a beverage. When you juice fruit, the fiber is removed, creating a watery sugar drink that overwhelms the pancreas and nervous system. You would not be able to eat the same amount of fruit as in a glass of fruit juice in one sitting. A small amount of juice that is diluted with water is a "better" choice. Most of the juices sold in the markets are quite far removed from real juice. The labels of most processed fruit juices say they are fruit beverages with some "real" juice added. This is way too much sugar for the body to effectively manage.

Soda is probably the most toxic beverage anyone can consume. Most of the ingredients found in soda were never even in the food chain. Sodas are carbonated with carbon dioxide gas. They have no nutritional value, contain high amounts of phosphates that contribute to bone loss and kidney damage, and contain tremendous amounts of white sugar and chemicals that can cause tooth decay and throw off the delicate balance of calcium and phosphorus in the body. This balance is crucial for optimal immune function and digestive health. When a can of diet soda is stored at room temperature, the aspartame in the soda breaks down into the chemical formaldehyde. Aspartame is the artificial sweetener found in most diet sodas.

A "better" alternative beverage is mineral water. It is still carbonated but doesn't have the chemicals found in soda. The "best" beverage to consume is good quality filtered spring water or herbal teas. There is a product called Techno that is a great coffee substitute; it's natural and a great way to eliminate caffeine and coffee beverages.

Coffee is a very addictive beverage. Coffee bars are the current hangout. But coffee has detrimental effects on the body. Caffeine is a stimulant, a drug. It produces an artificial lift. With repeated use it becomes less and less effective and more is needed to bring about the same level of stimulation. Eventually caffeine wears out certain cells in the pancreas by making them more sensitive and reducing their ability to quench the appetite. Caffeine has also been found to adversely affect the nerves by increasing the pulse rate, increasing the stomach's gastric secretions, destroying vitamin C, and stressing the kidneys, causing them to take excess salts from the blood.[7] Caffeine momentarily aids in weight loss, but over the long run it hinders weight loss because of the stress on the pancreas. Caffeine toxicity can cause weight gain, headaches, insomnia, nervousness, heart palpitations, and digestive problems. Many people also complain of these symptoms when trying to quit the caffeine habit. This usually doesn't last very long and is worth enduring for the health benefits of kicking the habit.

Finally, let's address salt. There is nothing wrong with salt. But as you might imagine, our commercial food industry found a way to make something wrong with it. Processed salt is known to contribute to heart and kidney disease, but sea salt is a wonderful source of nutrition. It has been shown to lower blood pressure and to reduce the risk of heart disease. Just the opposite is true of the regular product we find in saltshakers.

REDUCING THE STRESS LEVEL

For the most part, Janine was able to make these transitions without too much trouble. The only time she really exercised discipline in the past in the area of food was when she fasted. Although she knew the biblical reason for fasting, she also used it to trim off a few pounds here and there. In her heart she felt she was not being as effective an intercessor as she could be, and she knew her health distractions were definitely getting in the way. It was such a relief to know that many of her symptoms were triggered by her diet and her hormonal changes.

The only other issue she needed to address was REDUCING her stress level and getting a handle on her wayward emotions and occasional crankiness. She was now able to exercise the consistency and discipline to make the dietary changes that would facilitate permanent weight loss. This is a process that takes months to years. She didn't just wake up one day and "get discipline." In order to make it work, she had to commit her plans to the Lord on a daily basis and ask Him to lead her and guide her in every choice she made. It was clear that with the ups and downs of her emotions she needed God's loving mercy to show her what was hormonal and what was simply a bad attitude that needed to be dealt with.

This is more prevalent than we realize. Many women, especially Christian women, are tormented by the lack of control they feel over their emotions. Many resort to medications, while others simply suffer. As we take this issue before the throne of God's tender mercy, the Holy Spirit can reveal the emotions that are triggered by hormonal imbalances and those that are truly due to our unrepentant natures. This takes time and patience. But I have seen the faithfulness of God, and I know He changes hearts.

A crucial part of Janine's stress reduction was learning when to say no. She didn't want to offend or hurt anyone. She also felt it was her obligation as a pastor's wife always to be available. This was not only unrealistic but also unhealthy. As she learned to set healthier boundaries, she found that what she was able to give to her family, friends, and members of the congregation was quality help from a pure heart.

If you are facing menopause and feeling overwhelmed by the emotional changes, realize that God has not abandoned you. He still has a purpose for your life in spite of your feeling as if you're losing your mind. He will direct and guide you because He already has your steps ordered. If these words bring peace to your heart, pray with me, as we submit not only your hormonal balance to the Father's care but this great life transition as well.

Father, we know that not even one hair falls from our heads without your awareness. The changes in my body are not foreign to you, as you not only made every cell in my body but you also know how they are to func-

tion. I offer my body and all that I am to you as a living sacrifice. I ask you to give me discernment to know which part of what I feel is hormonal and which part is my own nature. Take my heart, create it anew, and help me to be disciplined in the changes I need to make to help this transition go smoothly. In Jesus Christ's name. Amen.

You made all the delicate, inner parts of my body
and knit me together in my mother's womb.

PSALM 139:13 NLT

Before I formed you in the womb I knew and approved of you [as My chosen instrument], and before you were born I separated and set you apart, consecrating you, and I appointed you
as a prophet to the nations.

JEREMIAH 1:5 AMP

FIT TIP #33:

REMOVE—Eliminate all processed foods from your diet, especially enriched grain products, products containing hydrogenated oils, canned fruit or vegetable products, juices, and processed soy items.

FIT TIP #34:

REPLACE—Add to your diet whole grains that are freshly milled or sprouted grain products, fresh expeller-press olive oil, flaxseed oil, and butter. Always choose the freshest foods possible.

FIT TIP #35:

REPAIR—If you are approaching or are already in menopause, con-tact a doctor or clinical nutritionist to support you in a healthy detox-ification program. The healthier your liver and digestive system, the easier menopause will be for you.

FIT TIP #36:

REDUCE—Implement a stress reduction program into your lifestyle. Daily prayer, fellowship with the Lord, and journaling are the most important aspects of any stress reduction program. Stress management will help reduce one of the most common causes of diet failure: using food to fill the void caused by pain or stressful situations.

FIT FOR ETERNITY

The Next Step

Although obesity does not rank in the top ten causes of death, we know that diet is responsible for most illnesses we suffer today and that obesity contributes to the diseases that do rank in the top ten. There are thousands of diets on the market. Whole sections at bookstores are devoted to weight-loss books. At the natural foods expo there are thousands of products that perpetuate the lie offered by vendors competing for your dollar—products that offer temporary solutions to a problem that needs long-term attention. You'll hear compelling and convincing arguments, usually from hired spokespersons, that exude what we think of as health and beauty. But we can't be fooled into thinking these things offer any real or lasting solutions.

As I have shared the lives of several different women, you may have come to the conclusion that the one diet change common to all of them is the only diet anyone needs to follow. How they reached their goals varied, but the goal is the same. Whatever we put into our mouths must beg this question: "Will this item I am about to consume produce health in my body or promote disease?"

If we eat foods that God designed, before they are corrupted and processed, as close as possible to the way He designed them, and if we don't allow our flesh to rule over us, we will have health, reach our ideal weight, and maintain it permanently. We want to eat *real food*—physically, emotionally, and spiritually—don't we? Just as we need physical nourishment, we also need spiritual and emotional nourishment. How many people realize that if they go to church only to be entertained or only pray to get something from God, they are not being nourished with God's *real food*? His *real food* nourishes, strengthens, and reproduces life within us on every level. It's time to *get real*. It's time to get honest with God and with each other.

> # Will this item I am about to consume produce health in my body or promote disease?

Do we have to do it all? Yes, but not all at once. We live in a time when every one of our senses is bombarded regularly with temptations, so we have to address every area. We are blatantly lied to through the media every day about what is good for us and how nine out of ten doctors agree. But I must admit I get pretty angry when I hear that gummy animal-shaped candy is the recommended choice for vitamins for kids, or worse, that ketchup is a vegetable choice in many public schools. Marketers have one goal, to get you to spend your money on their products. Whether that is a new weight-loss pill, a machine that will supposedly burn fat off your abs in seven minutes per day, or keys to double your income in a few weeks or less, there are no shortcuts. I repeat, THERE ARE NO SHORTCUTS! Spiritually, emotionally, and physically we must take the time to properly build a healthy foundation and structure in our lives. Sorry, but I've thrown my magic wand away. It was defective.

Now we basically know what normal is, what healthy looks and should feel like, and what food should be. The goal is not to be perfect but to continually strive (in a good way) to do better. We start by starting. I believe we can gauge how we are doing by the subtle signs our minds and bodies give us on a daily basis. Here are my criteria:

1. Do you wake up with energy?
2. Do you need a stimulant to get you going (e.g., coffee)?
3. Do you feel tired after meals?
4. Do you have aches, pains, and allergies?

5. Do you have a short fuse (easily irritated)?
6. Has your weight fluctuated by more than ten pounds over the past five years?
7. Do you like what you see when you look in the mirror?
8. Do you have peace and joy with yourself and with God?
9. Do you have a sense of purpose and meaning in your life?
10. Are you effective in your life, family, work, and witness as a Christian?
11. Can you put your head on your pillow at night and know if you die you will awaken in the presence of Jesus Christ?

The answers to these questions should tell you if you are healthy, happy, and living a balanced life. We all need a reality check now and then. As I said at the beginning of this book, I spent most of my life fighting with God over His management of my life. How many of you know that this is *not* the key to success and happiness? The goal of this book—as you may have gathered by now—is not to give you another formula for the perfect weight-loss diet, but to show you a way of living that will make *dieting* an obsolete word in your vocabulary.

We as the body of Christ must rise up and set a new standard. We look way too much like the world. We are to stand out, peculiar and extraordinary. I'm not suggesting we give up makeup, acrylic nails, or hair styling and wear shapeless robes, but I am suggesting that our focus be surrendered to the Lord. That's where it needs to start. It's time for us to leave the Shangri-La of our complacency and be about our Father's business. He has given each one of us unique and special gifts. You can be sure we will be held accountable for what we have done with these gifts. Second Corinthians 5:10 confirms: "For we must all appear and be revealed as we are before the judgment seat of Christ, so that each one may receive [his pay] according to what he has done in the body, whether good or evil [considering what his purpose and motive have been, and what he has achieved, been busy with and given himself and his attention to accomplishing]" (AMP). Our gifts are not only for us to enjoy this life and to accomplish our personal goals, though I believe we are to enjoy life and have goals, but more important, the gifts God has given us are for the purpose of reaching people with the Gospel.

In Mark 8, we see that Jesus had been ministering to the people for three days. He looked out and was aware that they had needs. He noticed and had compassion on them and did not want to send them home hungry. He asked

His disciples what food they had. He took what little they had and multiplied it to feed more than four thousand people. I believe this is how He works in our lives as well. He sees the needs of the people and has compassion and pity on them. He then says to you and to me, "What do you have?" I may have a few health tools and a computer to write a few tips. You may have a voice that is anointed or the ability to build homes or cook great meals. We all have some-thing. We all have a purpose. He asks us to give to Him what we have, and He in turn will multiply our little to meet needs. This takes our working with Him, trusting Him, listening to Him, and allowing Him to take what we have. That is sometimes painful at the moment. It may look like a door closing or an oppor-tunity fading. But, dear one, the path to power in our lives is to know the Lord, spend time with Him so that He can create more of His nature in us and reveal His purpose for us, and then to trust Him and His Word and surrender our lives as vessels for His use. This may be happening in our current jobs or voca-tions. We aren't all called to serve in developing countries. We are called to bloom right where we are planted. But one thing I can guarantee: If you are distracted with your weight, health, and self-image, you will not be able to fulfill this purpose. The Lord is saying to each one of us, "I've given you the tools; now go, because there is someone waiting to hear the Gospel from you. There is someone looking to see the Gospel in you and through you." As we seek first the kingdom of God, everything will be provided for everything we are called to do.

> You may have a voice that is anointed or the ability to build homes or cook great meals.

I pray that *Fit for Eternity* has awakened you and motivated you to focus attention on your health for a deeper purpose than simply to feel good, and that it has given you useful tools to truly change your life forever. Be encouraged, my sister. It's time to get busy. God has a beautiful and marvelous plan for your life. I am excited for you, and I know that as you trust Him and share these truths with your friends and loved ones, we can make a revolution. The beauty you can and will exude will far exceed what the world offers, because you will reflect the inner beauty of peace and holiness in God. True radiance is not found in a bottle. When someone looks at you and says, "What's different about you?" you can say, "I am getting fit for eternity." I pray that as Jesus looks to find someone to dine with, because He is hungry, that He will see you and me and be very satisfied with the fruit on our branches. Until next time—be fruitful, be fit, and be useful for the Master's purpose.

So whoever cleanses himself [from what is ignoble and unclean]—who separates himself from contact with contaminating and corrupting influences—will [then himself] be a vessel set apart and useful for honorable and noble purposes, consecrated and profitable to the Master, fit and ready for any good work.

2 TIMOTHY 2:21 (AMP)

FIT TIP #37:

Be aware of what comes into your mind and heart through your senses. Don't tolerate commercials or advertisements that lure you in and entice you to buy or indulge in something that is not good for you. Don't let the Enemy gain any ground.

FIT TIP #38:

Whatever you do, do it in love, with peace, knowing that your heavenly Father loves you and has a glorious plan for your life. Whether you are changing your diet, exercising, or simply becoming more aware of the imbalances in your life, put your focus on Him first.

FIT-TIP SUMMARY

FIT TIP #1:

Buy a journal—a pretty one, one you will enjoy picking up on a daily basis. When I see beautiful journals, I often buy them in bulk to share with others. There are so many choices. Each person has her own preference. Treat yourself.

FIT TIP #2:

The first truth to know is that God loves you and created you for a special purpose. On index cards, write out five truths from God's Word regarding His love for you. Post them everywhere: in your house, your car, or any place you frequent. Read these verses daily and allow God to renew your mind and begin to heal those wounded places where lies have reigned for so long.

FIT TIP #3:

Let your food cravings tell you what diet is best for you. A craving for sweets, coffee, fruits, and refined carbohydrates indicates a need to increase the protein and cut out the stimulants. A craving for salty and fatty foods indicates a need to increase the fruits, whole grains, low-fat dairy products, and vegetables and go easy on the animal protein.

FIT TIP #4:

Eat breakfast. If your cravings typically are for salty or fatty foods, have some fruit or whole-grain cereal for breakfast. If you crave sugars, pastas, and bread, have eggs cooked in butter or hard-boiled with a slice of whole-grain toast and some turkey sausage.

FIT TIP #5:

As long as nutritional needs are met, there are no good or bad diets—only the right diet for you. Don't allow yourself to be influenced by what the advertisements say is healthy.

FIT TIP #6:

When you blow it, and we all do, don't quit; make a decision to do better at your next meal. Remember, it's not how many times you fall down that counts but how many times you get back up and keep moving.

FIT TIP #7:

Follow the hunger scale with every meal. On a scale of one to four, one is being starved and four is feeling stuffed. Begin eating at two and stop at three. This will help minimize the triggers to overeat due to being starved and will minimize the digestive discomfort that results from overeating.

FIT TIP #8:

Take walks with God. Instead of being focused on yourself and your weight, let each day be an opportunity to pray for those you love, your neighbors, your city, or the nation. At the end of each walk, journal your thoughts and observations and watch what God will do.

FIT TIP #9:

Don't ignore your emotions and thoughts. Instead, put them to the test. If the feeling or thought is not based on God's truth as revealed in His Word, then find a Scripture to replace the lie. Write it on several cards and place them all over your house, car, and day planner. Anywhere you will see it, post it. Memorize the verses, and when the lie comes into your head, focus on the truth you know, and that truth will set you free.

FIT TIP #10:

Exercise in moderation. Some people benefit most from a brisk walk, while others like the exhilaration of a run on a path or on the beach. Weight training is an excellent way to tone and build muscle. Each person's body has different requirements. Listen to your body, and don't ignore the warning signals. Don't exercise if you are weak and tired. As you pay attention to your body's signals, tailor a workout that suits you best.

FIT TIP #11:

Be prepared. Never leave home without a plan for your meals for the day. As you plan your week, also plan your meals and snacks. If you know you have meetings or parties scheduled, plan around them so that you are never caught hungry and off guard out in the fast-food wilderness.

FIT TIP #12:

Don't buy any unhealthy snack foods. Keep your environment safe, healthy, and pure. Trust me, if it's in the house, you will eat it.

FIT TIP #13:

Make a list of restaurants that have foods on their menus that you enjoy and that are also healthy for you. When friends ask you out to lunch, ask them if they'd like to try someplace new.

FIT TIP #14:

Exercise your spirit and mind. Buy or make Scripture memory cards and cuddle up in a cozy spot with some relaxing instrumental music to meditate on God's Word, asking the Holy Spirit to make it come alive for you.

FIT TIP #15:

Exercise your body with low-impact cardiovascular, fat-burning exercises. Swimming laps is an amazing workout that really trims the fat. Set a goal for the amount of time you will swim and then focus on doing more and more laps in that time frame. Later on extend the time until you reach a comfortable yet challenging workout. Water aerobics are available for those who don't really care for lap swimming. Meditate on the Lord and pray as you swim.

FIT TIP #16:

Take a deep-breathing exercise class or look up information on how to breathe properly. Many excellent resources are available. In deep-breathing exercises, the focus is on effortless breathing. Don't force it; simply allow your body to relax. Perhaps you can imagine the Holy Spirit refreshing and renewing your body with His precious breath of life. Out with the old unhealthy habits and in with the new, which are only available by trusting the Father's path of life.

FIT TIP #17:

What did you learn about food from your parents? How was food used to celebrate in your home? Were you ever rewarded with food for good behavior? Were you ever sent away from the table for poor behavior? Journal what you learned about food from your childhood and note how these behaviors affect you now.

FIT TIP #18:

What did you learn about resolving conflict? How did your parents deal with their anger and frustrations? When you are angry, sad, frustrated, or hurt, do you eat, work, or shop? If none of these things, take some time to think about what you do when you experience these emotions, and journal your responses.

FIT TIP #19:

Take a moment out of each day and do a "body check" in which you pause and take note of how you feel, your posture, any tension in your neck or shoulders, any aches or pains, and do something about your observations. Whether that is standing and stretching, taking a walk, or having a cup of herbal tea, acknowledge your body and treat it lovingly, and it will continue to show you warning signs when they are still small and manageable. Perhaps your action step may be to call your doctor, but do something. Don't ignore the signals.

FIT TIP #20:

Take two hours and do the exercise described in chapter seven that will help you see yourself as God sees you. The Lord will lead you to seeing the false beliefs, repenting of them, and being filled with His truth.

FIT TIP #21:

Don't buy unhealthy snack foods. Keep your environment safe, healthy, and pure. For example, keep fresh or frozen berries or grapes on hand for a sweet snack. If it's in the house, you will eat it.

FIT TIP #22:

Take a trip to the grocery store and buy tasty, healthy foods. Based on what you can afford, start buying healthier ingredients to cook with. Maybe you can replace one unhealthy choice per week, maybe more. Whatever you are able to do, commit to it. For example, purchase sparkling water instead of soda, Stevia (a natural herbal sweetener) instead of your usual sugar substitute or frozen or fresh berries or grapes in place of ice cream.

FIT TIP #23:

Include your children in your "get healthy" campaign. Making them active participants educates them as well as reduces the stress of your doing it all on your own.

FIT TIP #24:

Make a meal plan and shopping list before you go to the store. This way you are less tempted to buy impulsively.

FIT TIP #25:

Start shopping at local farmers' markets. Many of the farmers offer produce free of pesticides and genetic modification. The prices are usually reasonable, and since the markets are usually set up outside, it's a good opportunity to get fresh air as well as experience shopping the way our ancestors probably did.

FIT TIP #26:

Exercise at or below your target heart rate for maximum aerobic efficiency. Use the 180-Formula to determine your maximum aerobic target heart rate.

FIT TIP #27:

Determine where you will eat your meals and create a healing environment for your senses. Play soothing music, have pleasant lighting, light scented candles. Use the "good" dishes and enjoy every aspect of every meal.

FIT TIP #28:

Count to twenty after each bite. Remember, it takes twenty minutes for your brain to notice your stomach is full. Take your time and relax.

FIT TIP #29:

Quit eating refined sugar. It's not good for you; you do know that by now, don't you?

FIT TIP #30:

Light weight lifting and mild cardiovascular exercise at least three times a week for no less than twenty minutes each time can help support and strengthen bone density. Speak to your physician and consult a personal trainer at the gym for exercises and limitations.

FIT TIP #31:

Develop an impulse strategy. When you crave sweets, know ahead of time what you will do about it. Whatever your vulnerable issue is, decide beforehand how you will manage it and tell your fitness accountability partner for added support.

FIT TIP #32:

Eat foods that are God-made. Buy fresh produce instead of canned. Canned foods have preservatives that are not conducive to life and health.

FIT TIP #33:

REMOVE—Eliminate all processed foods from your diet, especially enriched grain products, products containing hydrogenated oils, canned fruit or vegetable products, juices, and processed soy items.

FIT TIP #34:

REPLACE—Add to your diet whole grains that are freshly milled or sprouted grain products, fresh expeller-press olive oil, flaxseed oil, and butter. Always choose the freshest foods possible.

FIT TIP #35:

REPAIR—If you are approaching or are already in menopause, contact a doctor or clinical nutritionist to support you in a healthy detoxification program. The healthier your liver and digestive system, the easier menopause will be for you.

FIT TIP #36:

REDUCE—Implement a stress reduction program into your lifestyle. Daily prayer, fellowship with the Lord, and journaling are the most important aspects of any stress reduction program. Stress management will help reduce one of the most common causes of diet failure: using food to fill the void caused by pain or stressful situations.

FIT TIP #37:

Be aware of what comes into your mind and heart through your senses. Don't tolerate commercials or advertisements that lure you in and entice you to buy or indulge in something that is not good for you. Don't let the Enemy gain any ground.

FIT TIP #38:

Whatever you do, do it in love, with peace, knowing that your heavenly Father loves you and has a glorious plan for your life. Whether you are changing your diet, exercising, or simply becoming more aware of the imbalances in your life, put your focus on Him first.

DR. ROYAL LEE AND QUALITY NUTRITION

Dr. Royal Lee, a dentist, believed that you could change the function of the body by replenishing the nutritional factors that had been deleted from foods through processing. He was scorned, persecuted, and prosecuted as a fanatic due to his beliefs. In the 1920s he founded Standard Process Labs, Inc.

We have all benefited from the mind of Royal Lee. He invented the governor motor used on dental drills. But this is only one of his more than six hundred patents. His hobby was nutrition. He noticed in his practice of dentistry that his sophisticated, "civilized" patients had more dental caries (cavities) than simple farmers. He believed that the refined processed diet of "civilized" people was missing something essential for health. So he set his inventive mind and vast resources to attempting to solve the problem.

Dr. Lee bought quality farms and raised the foods to retain as many nutrients as possible. He maintained the farms with no pesticides or chemical fertilizers. He invented ways of bringing this quality to the consumer. Standard Process products are whole foods concentrated to therapeutic potency. They are very different from manufactured nutrients that can be purchased from health food stores. Many of them are synthesized from food or chemicals like coal tar or rancid oils.

In the 1930s Dr. Lee said that there were two primary reasons for the breakdown of health in our country: the refinement of grain and adulteration of oil. Recently a study conducted by the Harvard School of Public Health, authored by Dr. Walter Willett, showed some very interesting findings regarding heart disease.[1] This study looked at the diets of 90,000 nurses and concluded that the number one dietary indication of heart disease was the amount of margarine and other hydrogenated and partially hydrogenated fats consumed in the diet. What do you think was number two? It was none other than white bread and white flour products. In 1993 scientists proved what Dr. Lee believed in 1930. Yet the shelves of our grocery stores are stocked full of these and many other items.

PROCESSED VS. RAW MILK

When my parents were kids, milk was delivered to their homes and left on the front porch. It separated, with the cream rising to the top. If it was left out on the counter, it wouldn't spoil. Rather, the milk soured. When I was a kid, we no longer had milk delivered but purchased it from the big supermarket in the neighborhood. There was no cream on the top and it no longer came in glass bottles but in cardboard cartons. If it was left out it would spoil, and the smell was really awful. The cream was sold in a separate container for quite a hefty price. But what are pasteurization and homogenization? Maybe if we understood the process, we could make educated choices about drinking raw or pasteurized milk.

Pasteurization is a process that heats the milk to high temperatures to kill supposedly unwanted bacteria. This process came about at a time when many people were dying from tuberculosis. Louis Pasteur's germ theory seemed to be a solution to the woes that plagued a society fearful of dying from this dreaded disease. At the same time farmers were looking for solutions to help them not lose money due to the inability to process the milk fast enough. While Louis Pasteur's theories were widely marketed and accepted, they were just theories. The possibility of tremendous financial gain caused what little doubt remained to be swept under the carpet.

Several factors make raw milk a superior food to pasteurized milk, including the cleanliness regulations, the herd tests, the employee health examinations, and nutrition values. Raw certified milk is tested daily by a lab for the Certified Milk Commission for cleanliness;[1] pasteurized milk is tested only eight times per year by the health department. The raw milk herds are tested weekly by the County Medical Milk Commission for sanitation, whereas the pasteurized herds are inspected monthly. Employee health examinations for those who work with pasteurized herds occur at hiring and none thereafter. The raw milk herd employees are tested monthly at the certified farms as well as periodically for treptococcus to insure disease-free milk. Chest X-rays or skin tests for TB are required monthly. Lastly, the nutrition values in pasteurized milk reflect the destruction of all enzymes, the anti-stiffness factor, several amino acids, vitamin A, 38 percent of vitamin B, vitamin C, and much of the soluble calcium and fat content.[2]

Homogenizing milk is a process whereby the fat is broken down into smaller globules so that the cream no longer rises to the top. This is a process of violently shaking or agitating the milk so that the large fat globules present in the milk are shattered into tiny, irregular pieces. This shattering is so complete and so effective that the fat globules are unable to regroup and remain suspended in the milk. Unfortunately, since the fat molecules are so small, this process now allows fat molecules to get into places in the body that they shouldn't, causing unnecessary stress on the gallbladder, heart, and blood vessels.

END NOTES

Introduction
1. *National Vital Statistics Report,* Vol. 49, No. 12, October 9, 2001.
2. *Merriam-Webster* references all taken from http://www.m-w.com/home.htm
3. *National Vital Statistics Report,* Vol. 49, No. 12, October 9, 2001.

Chapter 2
1. Louis Rubel, M.D., *The GP and the Endocrine Glands,* 1959.

Chapter 3
1. These supplements are made by Standard Process Labs, Inc. I often recommend them in my practice. If you think you need such supplements, be sure you use them on recommendation of a health-care provider. Standard Process products are only available through licensed health-care facilities. If you look up their Web site—*www.standardprocess.com*—you can contact them for a practitioner near you.

Chapter 4
1. Hans Selye, M.D., *The Stress of Life* (New York: McGraw-Hill, 1956), 42.
2. Made by Standard Process Labs, Inc.

Chapter 5
1. Theresa Burke, Ph.D., *Forbidden Grief—The Unspoken Pain of Abortion* (San Francisco: Acorn Books, 2002).
2. Both made by Standard Process Labs, Inc.
3. Elliot Abravanel, M.D., and Elizabeth King Morrison, *Dr. Abravanel's Body-Type Diet and Lifetime Nutrition Plan* (New York: Bantam Books, Inc., 1999).
4. John Lee, M.D., *What Your Doctor May Not Tell You About Menopause* (New York: Time Warner, 1996), 34.

Chapter 6
1. J. H. Stein, J. G. Keevil, S. Aeschlimann, and J. D. Folts, "Purple grape juice improves endothelial function and reduces the susceptibility of LDL cholesterol in patients with coronary artery disease." *Circulation,* September 7, 1999.
2. H. Teragawa, M. Kato, T. Yamagata, et al., "The Preventive Effect of Magnesium on Coronary Spasm in Patients With Vasospastic Angina," *Chest,* December 2000, 118(6): 1690–695. (Address: Hiroki Teragawa, M.D., First Dept Intern Med, Hiroshima

University School of Med, 1–2–3 Kasumi, Minamiku, Hiroshima, Japan 734–8851.)
3. A special cold process that preserves the nutrients.
4. John Courtney, *Clinical Reference Guide*, 1996, 25.
5. While many of my colleagues do not find the *Eat Right for Your Type Diet* by Dr. Peter D'Adamo credible, I have noticed certain traits that are common in people of the same blood type (Putnam Son's, 1996). Dr. D'Adamo's book offers some sound nutritional advice that if followed closely will cause most people to notice a huge difference in their overall health. However, there is no one program that will work for everyone.
6. D. J. McNamara, "Dietary Cholesterol and Atherosclerosis," *Biochemistry Biophysics, 2000*; 1529:310–320.

Chapter 8
1. Henry Wright, *A More Excellent Way* (Thomaston, Ga.: Pleasant Valley Publications, 2000).
2. Virginia Worthington, "Nutritional Quality of Organic Versus Conventional Fruits, Vegetables, and Grains," J Alternative Complementary Med, 2001; 7(2): 161–73. #37809 (August 2001).

Chapter 9
1. Phil Maffetone, *In Fitness and in Health* (Stamford, N.Y.: David Barmore Productions, 1997), 72–73.
2. Corinne Netzer, *The Complete Book of Food Counts* (New York: MJF Books, Fine Communications, 1997).

Chapter 10
1. Nancy Appleton, Ph.D., *Lick the Sugar Habit* (New York: Avery Publishing Group, Putnam, 1996).
2. Melvin Page, D.D.S., *Health vs. Disease* (St. Petersburg, Fla.: The Page Foundation, 1960), 59.
3. K. Johnson, "Higher Protein Intake Can Avert Bone Loss," *Family Practice News*, November 15, 2000:7. 36488B.

Chapter 11
1. From Standard Process Labs, Inc.
2. Made by Metagenics.
3. SP Greenfood and Cataplex ACP by Standard Process Labs, Inc.
4. In my practice I use a product called Symplex-F, produced by Standard Process Labs, Inc.
5. Standard Process Labs makes an excellent source of chlorophyll called Chlorophyll Complex Perles.
6. Michio Kushi, *The Cancer Prevention Diet* (New York: St. Martin's Press, 1993), 116.
7. Melvin Page, D.D.S., "Coffee, Tea, Tobacco, and Alcohol," *Health vs. Disease* (St. Petersburg, Fla.: The Page Foundation, 1960), 67–68.

Appendix A
1. Dr. Walter Willett, "Intake of Trans Fatty Acids and Risk of Coronary Heart Disease Among Women," *Lancet*, March 6, 1993; 341(8845):581–5.

Appendix B
1. This information was gathered at a California dairy. Each state has its own standards. But there are national requirements.
2. AltaDena Dairy report on Raw Certified and Pasteurized Milk.